BLACK MEDICINE III

Low Blows

BLACK MEDICINE III

Low Blows

by
N. Mashiro, Ph.D.

Published by Paladin Press
Boulder, Colorado

Also by N. Mashiro, Ph.D.:

Black Medicine I: The Dark Art of Death
Black Medicine II: Weapons at Hand
Black Medicine IV: Equalizers

Black Medicine III:
Low Blows
by N. Mashiro, Ph.D.

Copyright © 1981 by Paladin Press

ISBN 13: 978-0-87364-214-9
Printed in the United States of America

Published by Paladin Press, a division of
Paladin Enterprises, Inc.
Gunbarrel Tech Center
7077 Winchester Circle
Boulder, Colorado 80301 USA
+1.303.443.7250

Direct inquiries and/or orders to the above address.

PALADIN, PALADIN PRESS, and the "horse head" design
are trademarks belonging to Paladin Enterprises and .
registered in United States Patent and Trademark Office.

Library of Congress Cataloging in Publication Data

Visit our Web site at www.paladin-press.com

TABLE OF CONTENTS

	Introduction	1
1.	Fistfighting	5
2.	Wrist Releases	25
3.	Escapes from Chokes & Lapel Grips	45
4.	Escapes from Headlocks	61
5.	Defense from the Ground	71
6.	Escapes from an Unfriendly Embrace	85
7.	Attacks from the Rear	91
8.	Defending Against Knives & Clubs	107

WARNING

The techniques outlined in this book are aggressive and violent and are *not* meant to take the place of qualified professional instruction. Attempting any of the techniques in this book could result in harm to life or limb. Therefore, this book is offered for information purposes only. Neither the author nor the publisher assumes any responsibility for the use of misuse of the information contained herein.

INTRODUCTION

The first two volumes in this series, **The Dark Art of Death** and **Weapons At Hand**, were intended to serve as exhaustive references on the vulnerable points of the human body, the body's natural weapons, and those common objects which can be pressed into service as makeshift weapons in an emergency.

The enthusiastic acceptance of these books by the martial community has been a source of great pleasure and pride to me, but readers have compained that the previous works did not discuss the all-important subject of *how* to use these weapons against an opponent's vulnerable areas. It is to this question that the present book (and the next one) must be addressed.

In my martial arts studies I have concentrated mainly on forms of karate, but with a very strong interest in that type of fighting commonly known as self-defense. Self-defense is a crude method of fighting, hardly an art at all, which is in every way inferior to any of the more sophisticated systems of hand-to-hand combat. It does have a single overriding virtue, though, which puts the others to shame. Self-defense techniques can be taught to novices in minutes, and if the novices are serious of mind and moderately sound of body, they can then perform the techniques with devastating effect.

By contrast, a karate student is shown how to punch during his very first lesson, but it may be years before he can deliver the lightning-fast, body-shattering punch which was once used for crashing through samurai armor. Some karate masters have studied the art for thirty years or more before

1

becoming satisfied that they have mastered this punch.

This is the difference between karate and self-defense. A highly trained karateist could fight a room full of self-defense students and might well defeat them all. Similarly, a well-trained self-defense student might well prevail against a room full of barnyard (untutored) fighters. A ten-hour course in self-defense, or even a two-hour tutorial, can make a helpless person relatively formidable against most opponents. Ten years of full contact karate lessons can make you formidable against nearly anybody. Ten hours of karate training does almost no good at all.

And there is another important difference: you can't learn karate from a book. Karate training involves a rigorous physical, emotional, and mental discipline which simply cannot be captured in the written word. For one thing, traditional karate derives much of its devastating speed from mental processes related to Zen Buddhism, concepts which can be understood by dedicated students but which cannot be expressed in words at all.

Whether or not self-defense can be learned from a book is an open question. Certainly the general public thinks it is possible, judging from the large number of self-defense texts littering the bookstores. Unfortunately, most of these books have been written by good fighters who are not good writers. They are written by athletes who have forgotten how little speed, strength, and agility is possessed by the average person. Some of the books have been written by persons who can only be described as pathologically deranged. Such persons would rather kill than wound, rather injure than escape. To kill a man for the crime of trying to punch you in the nose (as these people advocate) is neither civilized nor responsible behavior.

For these reasons, I have approached my own discussion of self-defense techniques with a pronounced sense of caution. I do not want to publish just another mediocre and unusable book, written by someone who does not need it for an audience which cannot understand it. I have tried to organize the material into natural families of techniques, each of which stems from a specific attack and begins with a specific, basic defense. The theory is that a student can amuse himself by practicing a variety of counters to an attack, but at the same time he is almost unknowingly repeating the motions of the fundamental reaction which may save his life. As an example, while practicing defenses against a knife attack the student is encouraged to try various disarming techniques, all of which begin with a defensive side step to get out of the path of the blade. In this situation the simple act of getting out of the way is far more likely to save the student's life than any fancy disarming trick. This side step is presented as an integral part of all the disarming techniques, insuring that even those students who will never master any one of the tricks will still repetitively drill on the single motion which might really help them.

Low Blows concentrates exclusively on the use of the body's natural weapons, and only rarely mentions the use of makeshift weapons. This is quite deliberate. The study of self-defense through the use of knives, sticks, clubs, and firearms is a topic which I reserve for advanced students. This is partly a prejudice on my part, having learned from experience that a student who has become proficient in barehanded fighting can subsequently learn weapon handling by second nature. The opposite, however, seems not to be the case. An exclusively weapon-oriented student seems to fall apart when required to fight unarmed. Therefore, I like to teach my students the bare-handed techniques first. The next volume of the Black Medicine series, called **Equalizers,** will explore the more advanced subjects of fighting using kitchen knives, Bowie knives, bayonets and other daggers, yawara sticks, batons, canes, staffs, flexible weapons, pistols, rifles, and shotguns. I hope that readers will enjoy experimenting with these self-defense techniques and will never actually have any practical need for them. Self-defense techniques are by nature dirty, crude, damaging, and painful. They are also very, very effective. Good luck.

N. Mashiro
April 1981

3

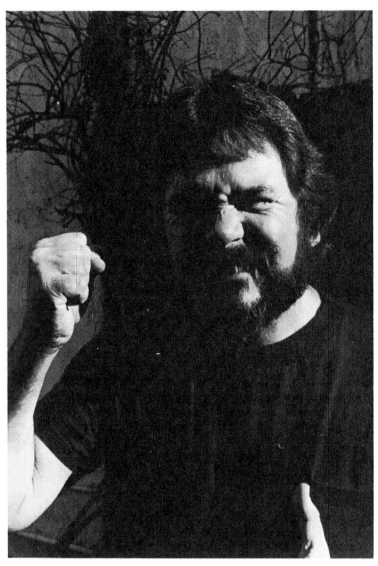

Figure 1: Everywhere you look, the ugly face of violence. Note the right arm cocked back ready to punch. This cocking motion is your signal to fight.

1. FISTFIGHTING

Fistfighting is the most common form of assault a man is likely to encounter, usually in the person of a demented longshoreman in a bar or an irate driver on the street. (Women have their own problems, which I will address later.) With a little nerve and determination a self-defense student can meet an attack from such a person with a reasonable probability of victory.

That doesn't mean that you can win every time—that only happens in Kung Fu movies. In my estimation a self-defense student has about a 50 percent chance of giving an assailant a severely painful surprise during the opening moves of a fistfight. The other 50 percent of the time you're going to get pounded like a tenderized steak. For most self-defense students, these 50-50 odds represent a substantial increase in their survival potential even if there is no guarantee of victory. If you want better odds than that you'll have to take up karate.

The key to success is the fact that most barroom brawlers and marauding motorists share a common failing: they're assholes. There are plenty of devastating ways to begin a fight, but these morons usually initiate hostilities with the old TV roundhouse punch. This attack is so common that you can actually anticipate it, guard against it, and if necessary you can use the punch as a wide-open invitation to dismember your opponent. That's where your chance to win lies. If the attacker uses a more sophisticated attack your victory or defeat will depend on luck, stamina, speed, and good sense. You will probably lose.

5

The first attack we'll consider is this typical right-hand, roundhouse blow to the face. Sometimes it comes as a punch, sometimes as a slap, but it always involves a fatal cocking of the elbow which can be the undoing of the attacker.

ATTACK #1

Right-hand roundhouse punch (or slap) to the face. The attacker scowls, twists his face into a mask of hate, snarls "I'll just have to teach you a lesson," pulls his right arm back in a dramatic wind-up, and then throws a punch as powerful (and slow) as a piledriver. (See Figure 1.)

BASIC DEFENSE #1

The first thing is to recognize that you may be about to be attacked. *Watch for that right-hand punch!* Think about your response and get ready. The instant his right arm starts backward to cock the elbow, you must start to move.

Take a deep step back with your right foot. This backward step pulls your face out of range of the incoming blow. Then use a left knife-hand block to meet the attack. The *knife-hand block* uses the little-finger edge of the palm to deflect the opponent's arm out to your left. From this basic position you can select from a wide variety of counterattacks.

The following list of eighteen counterattacks all begin from the basic defense position just described. Try out each of these possibilities in practice and then really work on one or two as your special weapons. Don't try to become proficient with them all. If you learn just one well enough to use it in a fight you won't need the others.

COUNTERATTACKS FOR SITUATION #1

1-1: You have just completed the block and your left hand is in contact with the attacker's arm. Grasp his right wrist with your left hand, pull on the arm lightly to straighten it, and then slap up under his elbow with your right palm (breaking his arm). Show this one to anybody who thinks that self-defense requires strength! This technique

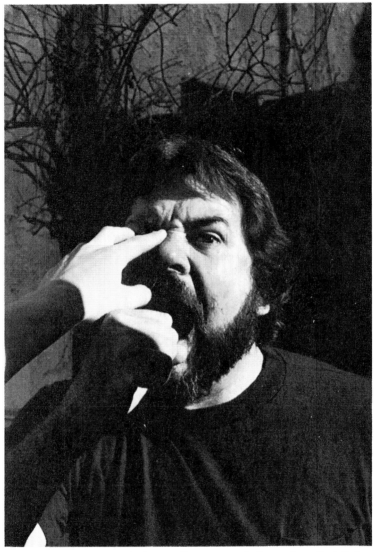

Figure 2: The typical roundhouse punch is so slow that it is a simple matter to lance your fingernails into the attacker's eyes before he can finish his swing. It's usually quite a surprise to him.

must be performed quickly to avoid the inevitable left-hand punch.

1-2: Parry the blow with the left hand as before, then straighten your left arm suddenly in a vicious stab to his eyes with your fingertips. The motion is like that of a striking snake, extremely fast. If you succeed in hitting the eyes you may blind the guy, so reserve this attack for situations which really require it. Even if you don't succeed in reaching his eyes, a near miss will shake him up and distract him. That gives you another opening. (See Figure 2.)

As a variation, try stabbing your finger tips into his eyes *without* blocking first! Most students can pre-empt this punch and end the fight with a lightning stab to the attacker's eyes. Try it! (For practice just try to tap your partner on the forehead—leave his eyes alone!)

1-3: Grasp his wrist with your left hand and pull him in as you stab your right finger tips into his eyes. This attack is similar to the previous one except that the right hand makes the eye-stabbing strike. It takes longer to do it this way, but some people prefer to use the right hand.

1-4: Grasp his wrist and pull him in as your right hand attacks his throat. Notice that there is a dynamic motion implied here. You pull him toward you so that he collides head-on with your outgoing blow. This can be a finger tip stab to the soft spot between the collarbones (possibly fatal) or a fist blow to the Adam's apple (also possibly fatal). Most people do not think of striking the throat due to watching countless TV heroes who always punch to the jaw. The throat is a large, soft, extremely vulnerable target which is not usually well defended. Practice a few attacks to the throat and see what you think.

1-5: Grasp his wrist and pull him in as your right hand delivers a karate chop to the left side of his neck. I don't normally advocate karate chops for self-defense students because it is hard to perform the cleaverlike blow correctly, but the side of the neck is so easy to hit and so vulnerable that even a completely inept blow there can produce significant results. Flatten out your hand, stiffen it up hard, and deliver the little-finger edge of the palm in an axelike motion against the opponent's neck, about three inches below the ear. If you succeed you'll make him dizzy at least. You may knock him out, and in rare cases you might just kill him. It's possible that the sight of a karate chop slicing through the air might give him second thoughts even if you don't hit anything . . . but it's better to hit!

1-6: If you don't feel comfortable with the karate chop, don't worry about it. Self-defense students can usually do as well or better using a hammer-fist blow (like pounding your first on a table). Smack him in the side of the neck with a right hammer fist. He'll reel on his heel.

1-7: Grab his wrist and pull him in as in the previous techniques, but deliver the chop or hammer-fist blow to the opponent's left temple about an inch behind the eye. You'll definitely give him a headache, you might knock him out, and if you are strong you could kill him. Be prepared for him to fall to your left due to the spinning effect of your combined pull and strike.

1-8: Grasp his wrist and pull him in as you strike up under the nose or the chin with a right palm-heel blow. I favor the palm-heel attack for self-defense students because they can hit with vicious enthusiasm without any danger of injuring their hands. A punch to the jaw may look easy in the movies, but I have found that untrained fighters almost always sprain their fingers or wrists when attempting to deliver powerful punches. (Try it out for yourself on a heavy punching bag and see.) That can be disasterous in a fight. The palm-heel attack uses the fleshy heel of the palm as a battering ram, immune to any injury, with which to inflict powerful blows on an adversary. The blow up under the chin is especially violent and can have fairly unpredictable results ranging from a bitten tongue to a broken neck.

1-9: Perform the usual basic defense and then deliver a right palm-heel strike to the solar plexus, which is the soft spot immediately beneath the breastbone. A sudden blow here will momentarily paralyze the opponent's diaphragm, knocking the wind out of him. There is also some chance of

9

doing damage to the stomach, liver, or spleen. An extremely powerful blow, delivered by a muscle-bound karate expert, can bruise the heart itself. The palm-heel attack can be used successfully against the abdomen and ribs, too, but the solar plexus is the most vulnerable target even if it is also the hardest to hit. Aim for it in the knowledge that a near miss may still do some damage. Note that some people have natural immunity to this attack due to strong abdominal muscles, deep layers of fat, extremely heavy clothing or high blood alcohol level.

1-10: A variation on the basic defense is to use the left knife-hand block to knock the incoming blow upward instead of sideways (an up-block). Then slide in close to the opponent, pushing his extended right arm up high over his shoulder. This will tighten and extend the ribs on his right side. Finish with a right palm-heel strike to the lowest ribs on the right side of his chest. You'll break them easily.

Unfortunately, this attack is a little more difficult to perform than the others and requires speed and good timing. (The other guy isn't going to just stand there and wait for you to get into position.) I have included it here mainly to show you another possible application of the palm-heel blow. It is every bit as useful as a fist punch.

1-11: Block normally, deflecting the incoming punch to the side, then slide forward and deliver a right rising elbow strike under the chin. The rising elbow strike is almost as useful as the palm-heel strike because it is extremely powerful, easy for a novice to use, and offers little possibility of injury to the user. Receiving an elbow strike under the chin feels like you've been hit with a club, and can easily result in a bitten tongue, broken teeth, broken or dislocated jaw, unconsciousness, or instant death due to spinal injuries. The disadvantage is that you have to get right in there to deliver it. Most people reserve the elbow blow for those times when circumstances have left you too close to the enemy to effectively use another technique. Don't deliberately take the time to step in close just to use your elbow. Also, don't neglect to use it when the range is appropriate.

1-12: Defend as usual, then slide in and deliver an elbow strike to the solar plexus (knocking the wind out of him, possibly killing him if you are very strong). Elbow strikes don't have to be traveling up to be effective. This one drives straight in under the rib cage, with a slight rising motion during impact. Performed correctly, the tip of the elbow penetrates deeply under the breastbone. To the receiver this feels like having the end of a broomstick rammed into his gut.

1-13: Step back and block as usual, then deliver a right shovel kick to the opponent's testicles. A shovel kick is the easiest karate kick to perform, and consists of pointing your toe toward the floor and then smacking the flat top of your foot up under the enemy's crotch. The "V" of his legs will automatically serve to guide your foot to the target, so all you have to do is punt. If your distance is off you will still hit him with the toe of your shoe, the top of your ankle or your shin. All are damaging.

1-14: It sometimes happens that your initial step back does not even begin to match the attacker's step forward. In this case you wind up nose-to-nose with him after your block. To get control of this situation, bring your right knee up smartly into his groin.

I should mention, however, that the old knee-to-the-groin trick taught by countless fathers to countless daughters does not work very well. Countless fathers also teach countless sons how to avoid getting hit there! The attack has to be fast and has to come as a complete surprise or it will not work.

An amusing variation you should learn goes like this. Suppose that you try to knee him with your right knee, but he does the natural thing and pulls his left thigh up across his groin to protect it. This will effectively nullify your attack unless you are a karate master and can put enough force into the blow to break his thighbone. (It can be done.) Your response should be to instantly put your right foot back down on the ground and snap your left knee into his groin. Try it gently with a practice partner and you will find that

11

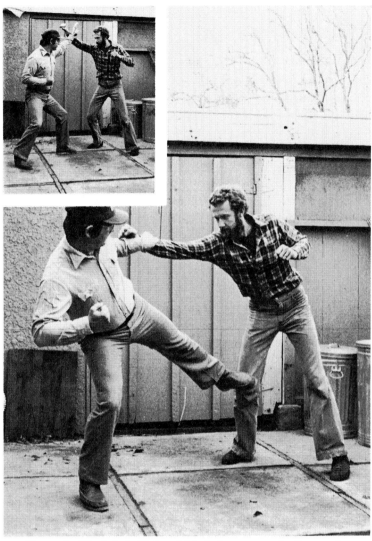

Figure 3: The left knife-hand block is common in the movies . . .
one of the few movie techniques which really works. The follow-
through, where you grab the attacker's arm to keep him off balance—
and then stamp on his knee to break it—are not so frequently seen.
Movie directors don't like this kick because it ends the fight too quickly
and takes one of the villains out of the story for weeks. Serious fighters
love it.

the thigh block can frequently be circumvented by switching feet this way. Be sure to guard your own groin at the same time.

1-15: Perform the basic defense (step back and block) as before. Then shift your weight back on your right (rear) foot and deliver a left side-thrust kick to the attacker's leading knee. The side-thrust kick to the knee is easy to perform. Just think of leaning a stick of kindling against a wall and then breaking it by stamping your foot against the middle of the stick. Everyone has done something like this at one time or another. The only difference is that instead of a stick of wood you are stamping on the enemy's leg at the knee. The results are about the same. (See Figure 3.)

The knee is a preposterous joint in which two long, strong bones are held together by several sets of small ligaments. Heavy pressure against the front or side of the knee when it is straight will easily rip these ligaments out by the roots, breaking the knee. Take care, though. This is not an injury which heals well. The person you do this to will be crippled permanently, so save it for the guy who really deseves it.

1-16: This technique presumes that the attacker steps forward into his punch with his right foot, putting his right knee within easy reach of your left foot. (Stepping forward with the right foot is fairly common but does not always happen, especially in practice where your partner may be "attacking" with stiff, unnatural motions.) As the punch comes in step back, block, and shift your weight to the right foot as before. Hook your left foot around the outside of his right knee so that the arch of your foot curls around to the back of the knee joint. In this position you can pull his knee forward, bending it, and then you can put your weight on your left foot and drive his bent knee powerfully into the floor. Depending on how hard you drive his knee into the ground you may simply humiliate him or you may shatter his kneecap, inflicting a very serious and long-lasting injury. (See Figure 4.)

If all has gone well, your opponent should now be kneeling on one injured knee directly in front of you. Let me

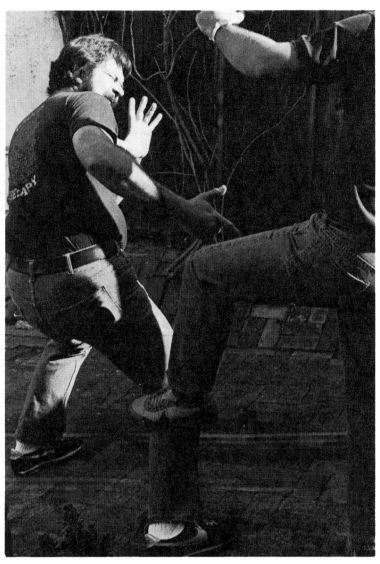

Figure 4: Stomping on the back of the opponent's knee is very effective because it is painful, unexpected, sudden, and it completely destroys the man's stance and mobility. It puts his head in reach of your knee, too.

point out two things about this position. First, notice how easy it is to use a hammer-fist attack to his face, skull, or neck. You may also be able to use a knee to rearrange his face depending on his exact landing position. Second, notice how easily he can attack your groin or grab your legs from his position below and in front of you. Better keep that in mind.

This technique is not always appropriate (his foot may be in the wrong position) but when circumstances are right it can be irresistible. The takedown is fast, painful, and very surprising. Best of all, when properly done the opponent can't run very well afterwards. That's all you need for a clean getaway.

1-17: Now and then I teach my students techniques intended for display to relatives. For some reason relatives want to believe that you aren't really learning anything useful in your self-defense class! (They feel threatened, I guess.) The following technique falls into this class. Use it when your brother wants to see some "self-defense." Don't us it in a fight unless you feel very confident of your ability.

Meet the incoming punch with the same basic defense as before, but angle the block to deflect the opponent's fist upward. Duck down low, slide under his arm to the outside and throw him by hooking your bent right arm under his right leg while striking upward under his chin with your left fist. As his head goes back your right arm lifts his leg and he topples over backwards. (For sake of demonstration, push gently up under your brother's chin with the palm of your hand. Don't clout him unless that's what you really want to do!)

ATTACK #2

So what happens if *the attacker leads off with his left fist,* like a boxer would? This isn't such an unlikely possibility, and after the 50 percent of all attacks which start with ride-side haymakers, left jabs come next in frequency. I train my students to be right-side specialists because they usually don't have the time (or the ability) to shift from right- to

15

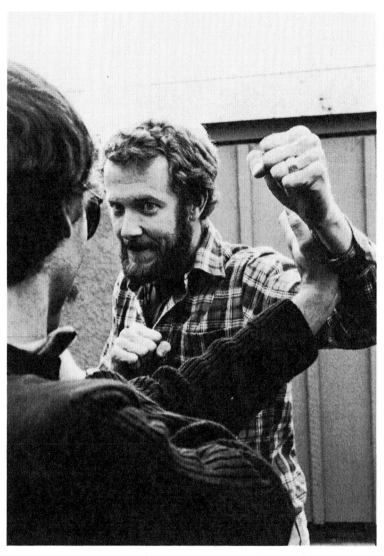

Figure 5: With the palm block you can deflect a left-hand punch and still be ready for the following right. This technique lets superficially trained self-defense students concentrate on defending against right-hand attacks only.

left-side defenses in mid-punch. Therefore I train them to parry the left hand and wait for the inevitable right-side attack.

BASIC DEFENSE #2

Step back with the right foot, and use a left palm-block to deflect the incoming punch. A palm-block is a solid, snappy slap. The idea is to slap the attacker's incoming left jab to your right so it misses your head, but not so much that you can't recover in time to meet his right hand if it is coming in next. (See Figure 5.)

COUNTERATTACKS FOR SITUATION #2

2-1: The best idea for a self-defense student is usually to block but don't counter. Just wait for the right hand strike and deal with it instead.

2-2: If you would rather strike back, not wait for a right-side attack, use the left palm-block as before and then slide in as you deliver a left knife-hand strike to the left side of his neck. Alternately, use a left hammer fist against the left side of his neck or temple.

Note that this is intended to be a coil-recoil motion. As you block your body twists to your right, then recoils suddenly to the left during the counterattack. This can be a very fast and powerful attack. Don't use it unless it feels very natural to you.

2-3: The palm-block used here is essentially a slap which hits the attacker's wrist and drives it out to your right. If your right hand slaps the back of his elbow to the left at the same instant you will dislocate or break his arm.

ATTACK #3

Right-hand punch (or slap) to the face. This is the same as attack #1, but the defensive response is different.

BASIC DEFENSE #3

Some students find that stepping back with the right foot feels awkward and unnatural for them. They would rather defend by stepping back with the left foot instead. Others would prefer to block with their right hands, apparently because they feel that the right hand is stronger and more coordinated. Since I try to use a student's natural inclinations to advantage, this section presents a few left-foot, right-hand defenses for these people.

There is an advantage to stepping back with the left foot in that you can then use a right hammer-fist blow as a block, a very powerful technique. Take a deep step back with your left foot, using the right hammer fist to meet the attack. A hammer fist applied to the soft inner side of an opponent's wrist can bruise nerves or actually break his arm.

COUNTERATTACKS FOR SITUATION #3

3-1: After connecting with the hammer block, raise your right fist slightly and deliver a hammer blow down on top of the opponent's right collarbone (breaking it). This is a sure way to end the fight, but there is a slight possibility of causing a fatal internal hemorrhage.

3-2: After connecting with the block, strike the opponent on the right side of his neck with a right knife-hand strike or a hammer fist. This blow will probably just make him dizzy, but again there is the possibility of a more serious injury in rare cases.

3-3: After delivering the block, duck down, slide in toward the opponent and strike him in the ribs with your right elbow (breaking the floating ribs and/or knocking the wind out of him). In this attack you are assumed to be at close range, as if he practically ran you over when you stepped back. Your right shoulder should be only inches from his chest. Bring your right arm down across your abdomen and point the elbow at the opponent's lower ribs or solar plexus. Now drive the sharp point of your elbow deeply into his body. You can hit harder if you use your left hand to push on your right fist as you strike.

3-4: After completing the block shift the weight to your left (rear) foot and deliver a right side-thrust kick to the opponent's knee, thigh, groin, or abdomen. This technique

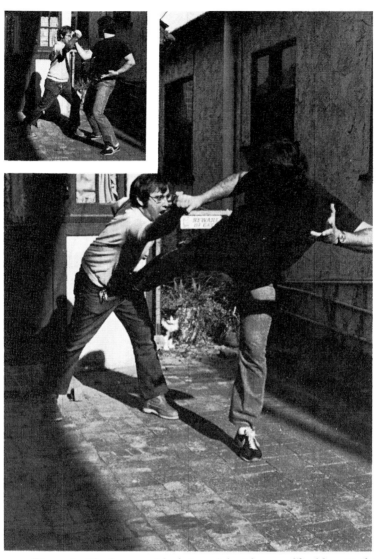

Figure 6: The hammer block is a violent hammerlike blow to the inside of the attacker's forearm which can stun nerves or even break bones. If you are fast you can also grab the opponent's (broken) arm and pull on it while you crush his bladder with your foot.

19

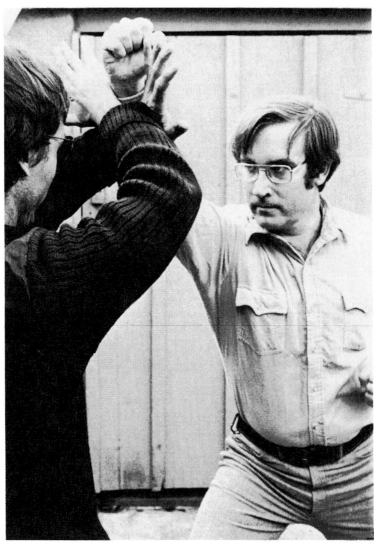

Figure 7: The "X" up-block is difficult to perform effectively but self-defense students like it because of the dramatic counterattacks it makes possible.

assumes that there is sufficient distance between you and your opponent to allow you to kick. The knee is by far the best target. Aim higher only to impress your friends during demonstrations. (See Figure 6.)

The next few fist-fighting techniques are not as simple to perform as the previous ones. They are presented for enrichment (for fun), and for use by those advanced students who have the inclination to master them. Although some of these tricks are flashy, they are also very risky. Use them when you choreograph the high school play, not when things get serious.

ATTACK #4

Right-hand punch (or slap) to face. This is the same attack as in the previous situations. It is the defensive response that is different.

BASIC DEFENSE #4

Step back with the right foot using an "X" up-block to parry the attack. The "X" up-block is formed by making fists, with the hands palm down and the right wrist crossed over the left one. This forms the "X" which is used to catch the opponent's incoming punch and deflect it upward. When performed properly, the "X" block can actually trap his arm, giving you a split-second chance to grab his wrist and work mischief with it. (See Figure 7.)

Remember, *these techniques are presented for your entertainment, not for practical use.* Don't try them in combat unless you are very sure of your ability to use the "X" block effectively. It is not easy.

4-1: Step back and use the "X" block to trap his arm momentarily. Use your right hand to grasp his wrist, then pull it sharply down and back toward your right hip. Press against the back of his elbow with your left forearm to control him. This produces pain in the arm but no particular damage to the opponent's body.

The basic idea here is to get his arm straightened with the back of the elbow on top. Rest the bony ridge of your left

21

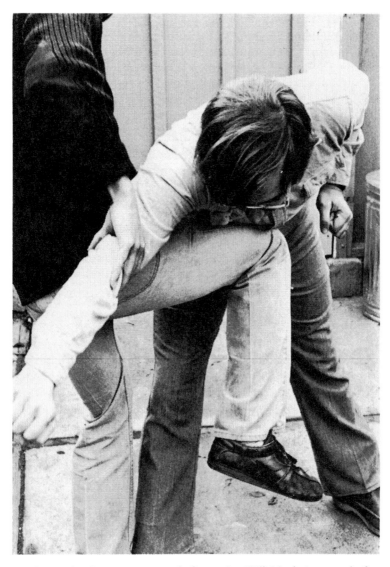

Figure 8: One counterattack from the "X" block is to grab the attacker's arm and jerk him down past your right hip as you lift your knee.

wrist against a spot about an inch above his elbow (your practice partner will tell you when you have the right spot). This brings pressure against the radial nerve (the funny bone nerve) and produces severe pain with very little effort on your part.

4-2: Do exactly as described in the previous technique, but deliver a left hammer blow to the back of his elbow to painfully dislocate the joint.

4-3: Grasp his wrist as before, then pull down and back really suddenly so he bends over at the waist. Finish with a left hammer blow to his kidney. The spot is about six inches up from the belt and two to three inches to either side of the spine. This is an extremely painful blow which can cause serious internal bleeding in some cases.

4-4: Grasp his wrist and yank it down past your right hip as described before. As the opponent starts to fall forward off balance, shift your weight to your left foot and bring your right knee up smartly into his chest. Your continuing pull on his arm will greatly magnify the force of the impact. A collapse of the cardiopulmonary system is a possibility here, due in part to a crushed rib cage. This is a very powerful attack even for a novice. (See Figure 8.)

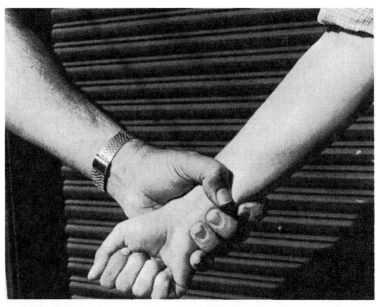

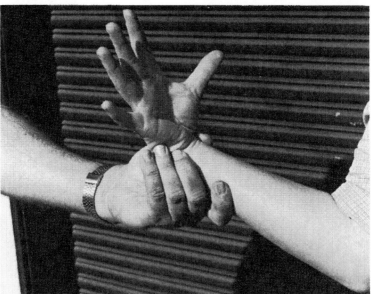

Figure 9: The classic wrist-release technique consists of twisting your hand up and out against the opponent's thumb.

24

2. WRIST RELEASES

Envision a situation where someone is trying to limit your movements by holding your wrists. This could be any friendly or unfriendly situation, like having a few friends trying to hold you down to tickle you, or having a mugger trying to drag you into a dark alley. The ability to quickly and surely escape when your wrists or arms have been grasped is basic to any self-defense student's training.

The lack of such training can be very embarrassing to a martial artist. I recall a karate black belt who was grabbed by some friends and thrown into the ocean as a joke. He remarked later that he could have killed them easily at any moment, but he couldn't make them let go without injuring them! Since it was just a playful joke he had to let himself be dunked. A self-defense student might not always be able to kill with his bare hands, but he'd better be able to perform an effective wrist release!

The important thing, remember, is to get loose. If the situation is serious and you can incidentally maim, mutilate, and massacre the other guy as you escape so much the better. But be satisfied if the technique results in your freedom. Don't press your luck beyond that point without a very good reason.

ATTACK #5

Your right wrist has been grasped by the opponent's left hand. Usually this puts the palm of his hand against the back of your wrist with his fingers curling under your arm and his thumb on top. He then tries to hold you against your will or to drag you off in some direction where you don't want to go.

BASIC DEFENSE #5

To get free, twist your wrist in his grip until the narrow upper edge of the wrist is against his thumb. This is the weak part of his grip. Use a circular motion to pull your hand toward the center of your body, then up to shoulder level, and then out and down to your right. Make a complete, snappy circle and your wrist will pry itself free between his thumb and fingers. (See Figure 9.)

The key to success is to use your forearm as a pry bar, putting irresistible pressure against the tip of his thumb. There are very few men with hands strong enough to resist this simple release when performed by a person of average strength. Even these men can be overcome by some additional steps.

COUNTERATTACKS FOR SITUATION #5

If a simple escape isn't dramatic enough for you try one of these techniques instead.

5-1: Twist your hand counterclockwise in his grip until your palm is vertical (thumb down). From this position you can curl your fingers up over the top of his wrist. Grasp his wrist tightly. At this point your "imprisoned" hand is on top holding the attacker's wrist, while the attacker's hand is on the bottom still gripping your wrist. Clamp his fingers against your arm with your left palm so he cannot let go even if he wants to.

Now comes the fun part. Use the strength of your shoulders to twist his arm violently clockwise. This will spin him around with his back toward you and his arm twisted up in a knot over his left shoulder. Finish by yanking the arm straight down toward the floor (dislocating the shoulder) or by delivering a knee kick to the base of his spine (breaking the coccyx). (See Figure 10.)

5-2: This technique sounds preposterous but it really works well. The attacker is holding your right wrist in his

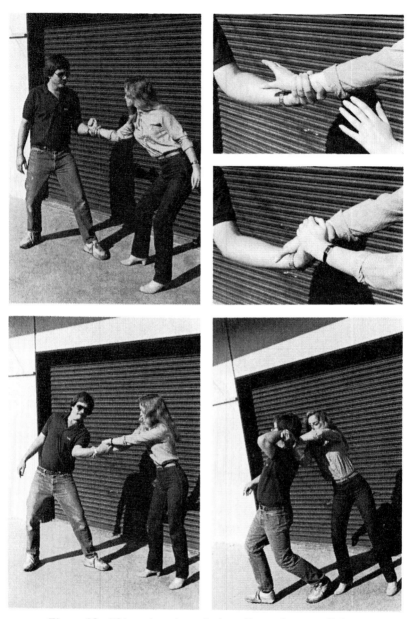

Figure 10: This wrist release isn't really a release at all, but an unexpected counteroffensive. The victim uses her hands to grab and lock
down the attacker's left hand, then twists it violently to her right.
Performed with sufficient conviction, this move will force the attacker
to spin around on his heel into a very uncomfortable position.

27

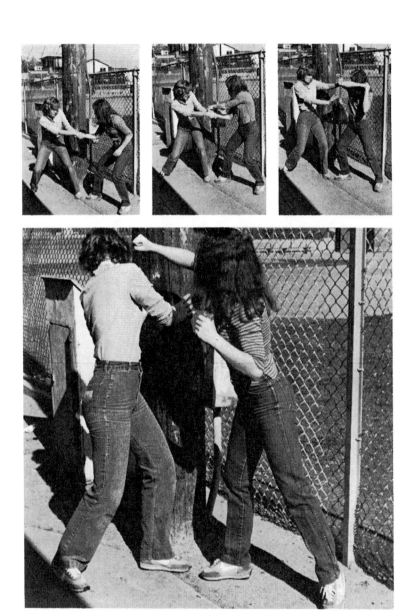

Figure 11: Another classic wrist release consists of grasping your captured hand with your free one and using the strength of both arms to tear your wrist free. The standard retaliation is a hammer-fist strike to the head.

left hand as before. Turn and take a short half-step to your left with your left foot, followed by a deeper step through to the left with your right foot. As you make the second step, point at an imaginary object in the distance with your captured hand. Be sure to push your right elbow into contact with his left elbow as you turn and point. When the elbows touch your hand will come free from his grip. As you feel your hand slipping out of his grip squat down slightly and deliver a back elbow strike to his abdomen (breaking ribs or knocking the wind out of him).

5-3: For that special surprise, don't try to get loose at all! Step in toward him and drive the captured hand up in a palm heel strike to the chin. Or jab at his eye. Your hand will come loose from his grip as you strike. This attack usually succeeds quite well because the opponent suffers from the assumption that your hand is under his control. He can't believe the captured hand is coming up to hit him until too late.

ATTACK #6

Your right wrist is grasped by both of the opponent's hands. Usually this means that his thumbs are across the top of your wrist and his fingers are firmly clenched around the lower side of your arm. This is a more difficult situation to deal with than the previous one.

BASIC DEFENSE #6

Reach down between his arms with your left hand and grasp your own right fist. Use both arms to pull the tangle of hands up and back toward your left shoulder, using your right forearm as a pry bar against the opponent's thumbs. In most cases you will be able to pry your arm free immediately.

COUNTERATTACKS FOR SITUATION #6

6-1: Perform the basic defense as described above. As your wrist comes free, retaliate with a right hammer blow to the face. Be sure to note the coil-recoil nature of the motion. You coil to the left as you pry your arm free,

29

and then recoil to the right to put added force behind the hammer-fist blow to the face. (See Figure 11.)

6-2: If you can't seem to pry your arm loose, don't lose hope. If the attacker is so foolish as to immobilize both of his hands while holding only one of yours, go ahead and hit him with your free hand. A hammer blow to the nose might be a very effective distraction. I guarantee that he'll let go of your wrist with at least one hand as soon as you start raining blows on his face, jabbing at his eyes, or kicking his knees. The instant he does, *move!* That's your golden chance to free your hand and get out of there.

ATTACK #7

Your right wrist is grasped by the opponent's right hand. This looks like a perverted handshake where the opponent deliberately bypassed your open hand and grabbed your wrist instead. It's a common trick.

BASIC DEFENSE #7

As always, use your forearm as a pry bar to put pressure against his thumb. In this case push your arm down slightly and then snap it up in a tight counterclockwise circle around his hand. After your wrist passes over the top of his hand you will see that he is losing his grasp on you. You can make the movement more forceful by completing the circle with a little body weight added to the strength of your arm on the downstroke.

COUNTERATTACKS FOR SITUATION #7

Here are two methods of doing more than simply getting free.

7-1: Perform the basic defense as described above. Then, as your right arm comes free give him a short, sharp punch to the testicles. Don't bother with hitting him in the stomach; put your fist where it counts. For those of you who are using palm-heel strikes instead of punches, turn your hand palm up and rake the heel right down his zipper and through to the back. He'll get the message. You didn't like having your arm held! (See Figure 12.)

30

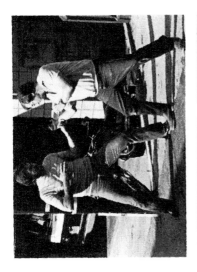

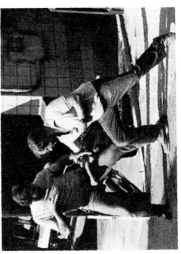

Figure 12: More experienced fistfighters will occasionally grab the opponent's wrist and use the hold to some advantage. One response is to twist free against his thumb and in the same motion punch straight to his groin. (This has to be fast, though, since he's just aching to use that free right hand and your face is awfully close . . .).

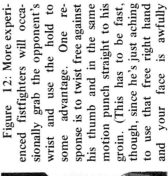

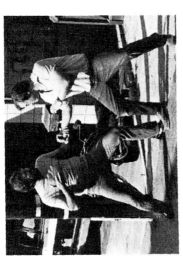

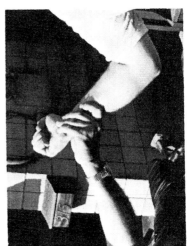

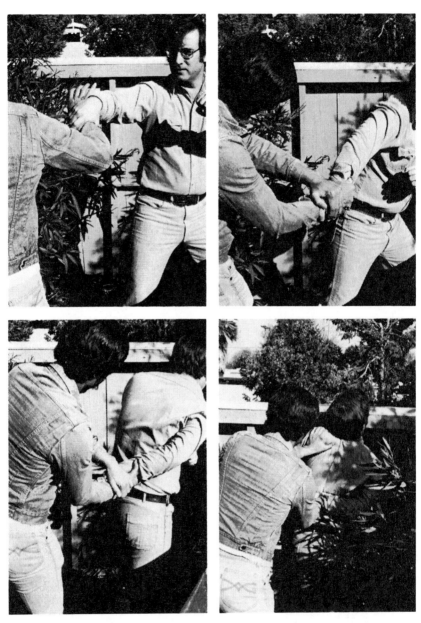

Figure 13: When your fistfighting opponent uses his leading hand to grab yours, you can pin his hand and twist him around into a hammer lock. Be careful, though, since he may know how to escape from a hammer lock (see Figure 38 for the end of this sequence).

32

7-2: This technique is similar to 5-1. Twist your hand counterclockwise in his grip until your fingers can reach up around the outside of his wrist to grasp it. Your hand must pass under his wrist so that the fingers can curl up the far side with the little finger leading. Clamp his fingers against your forearm with your left palm (so he cannot escape) and twist his arm violently clockwise. This will spin him around into a hammer lock. Finish with a knee kick to the coccyx or a shovel kick up into the groin from the rear. He'll never see it coming. (See Figure 13.)

ATTACK #8

The opponent grasps both of your wrists from the front. This means that he is holding your right wrist in his left hand and vice versa. Notice that this is really a neutral stance, since as long as he holds on to your wrists neither one of you can do anything with your hands.

BASIC DEFENSE #8

First try a simple one-hand release such as basic defense #5. Just because he elected to grab both of your hands doesn't mean that you have to free them both at once. Free one, then the other.

If you find that you don't have much success getting one hand free, try bringing your hands together to the point where your left hand can grasp his left wrist. Hold his wrist firmly while you twist your right hand free. Immobilizing his hand makes the escape much easier to work. (See Figure 14.)

COUNTERATTACKS FOR SITUATION #8

8-1: The next three counterattacks form a natural group, each beginning with a sudden motion which spins the opponent around on his heels. Although this technique is a little difficult to coordinate at first, and although an alerted practice partner can frustrate it easily, you will find that it works very effectively against a surprised opponent. Believe me, he'll be surprised.

Free your right wrist by twisting out against his thumb

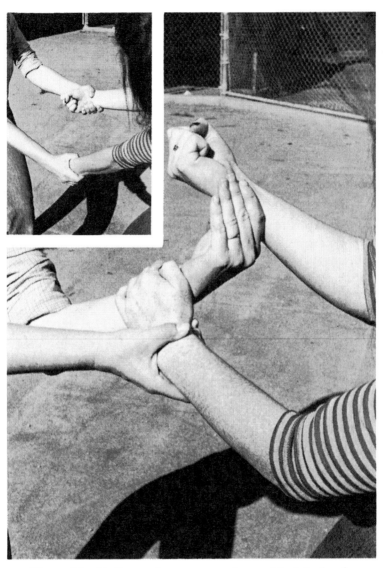

Figure 14: At times when someone has grabbed both of your wrists the easiest way out is to use one of your hands to help free the other.

(using basic defense #5 or #8). Now cup your right hand as if to drink water from it. Notice that the hand forms a natural hook when held in this position. Swing your left arm slightly out to your left to pull his right arm a few inches away from his body. Then swiftly hook him under the right armpit with your right hand. Your wrist will hit him in the armpit and the hook of your fingers will catch around the back of his shoulder or upper arm. Don't grab him, just hook his arm. Grasping takes too long, but hooking his arm with your cupped hand can be accomplished with blinding speed.

The next step is to give his shoulder a short, sharp, and very powerful yank to your right. Use your torso to provide the strength for this pull, not your arm alone. The idea is to suddenly spin him around at least a quarter turn. It sounds difficult but if the pull is extremely sudden it really works well. In one self-defense class demonstration I used this spin on an unsuspecting assistant and actually spun him completely around like a top, which surprised us both and ruined the point I was trying to make to the class.

As your opponent is spinning on his heel with that welcome look of shock on his ugly face, you will find that it is very easy to twist your left hand out of his grip using basic defense #5. While he is turning just swing your left hand across in front of your body and up in an arc to your left shoulder. You will be amazed at how naturally your wrist glides out of his hand while his brain is preoccupied with catching his balance.

If all has gone well, your opponent should now be standing with his right shoulder toward you. Grab the hair at the back of his head with your left hand and yank it straight down (not backwards) to drop him on his back. If the hair is too short to grab, reach over the top of his head and get a hold by digging your fingers into his eye sockets. Yank his head straight back so his face points toward the ceiling. To make the fall more violent throw your feet out from under you and drop on your chest, letting your weight drive his head down. He will fall violently straight down on the back of his head, with feet and arms flying in all directions. (See Figure 15.)

8-2: A variation of technique 8-1 is to spin the opponent all the way around with his back toward you and catch his neck in a strangle hold. Jerk him violently into the spin and then just let your right arm encircle his neck as he turns. Rest your left elbow on top of his left shoulder, and grasp your left bicep with your right hand. (Your little finger fits into the fold of the elbow.) Place your left hand on the back of his head and grasp the hair there if you wish. To apply the choke hold, force his head forward with your left hand while you pry the bony edge of your right wrist back into the center of his throat just under the jaw.

This choke is an attack on the windpipe and is extremely dangerous and painful. A violent application of this hold can sprain or even break the opponent's neck. An inexpert application of the strangle hold is worse than no hold at all. While using such a hold you may be very vulnerable to a variety of throws and counterblows. The victim will become extremely agitated as soon as he feels the pain, and will attempt the most desperate countermeasures. If you are not willing to take the soldier's way out (snapping the neck) it may take from five seconds to two *minutes* to subdue the opponent. It could be a lengthy struggle.

8-3: A variation of the strangle hold described above is the carotid artery hold (called "the sleeper"). I find it more useful and less dangerous (to everyone) than the strangle hold.

Encircle his neck as before, pinching his throat in the bend of your arm. Hook your hands together on top of his left shoulder, and anchor them in place by pressing your left forearm tightly down his back. Squeeze the neck (just beneath the jaw) between your bicep and forearm to close the carotid arteries. Be sure to tuck your head down so he can't make a sudden stab back over his shoulder with his finger tips and put out your eyes!

This cuts off the supply of blood to the brain and produces unconsciousness in seconds. Holding this position for several minutes will produce severe brain damage or death. There is relatively little danger of damage to the

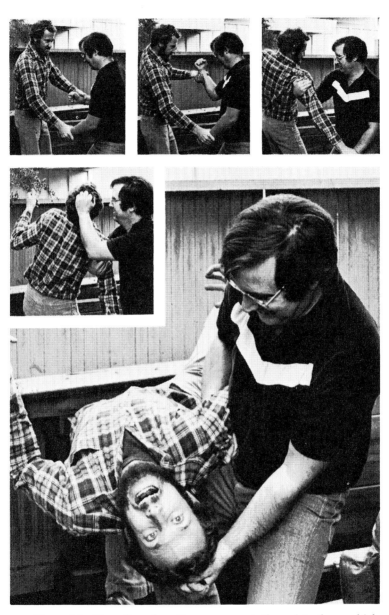

Figure 15: One of my favorite maneuvers is the wrist release which suddenly becomes a spinning takedown. The motions required are complex, but with a little practice this technique is fast as lightning.

spine or the trachea from this hold, and it is not especially painful.

This hold is the magical attack which TV scriptwriters have sought for years, in which the victim passes out immediately and awakens as good as new a few minutes later. Unfortunately, the TV heroes usually pistolwhip the victim over the head or chop him on the back of the neck to produce this "anaesthetic" effect. Do not be deceived. Such attacks are frequently lethal, and carry with them the possibility of crippling brain injury if the victim is not fortunate enough to die immediately. People do not wake up smiling ruefully after being brained with a heavy pistol. Even this relatively safe judo hold can be dangerous if something goes wrong.

8-4: This technique is for those of you who cannot master the shoulder-spin described in the preceding paragraphs. Twist your hands in his grip and grab his wrists (similar to techniques 5-1 and 7-2). Pull his hands out to the sides and alternately butt him in the face with the top of your head and kick him in the groin until he submits. The beauty of this combination is that the blow to the face makes him throw his head back and his hips come forward. The kick makes him jerk his hips away which brings his face back into range again. With good timing you can get him rocking like a seesaw! Note that it is not really necessary to grasp his wrists since you can use his grip on you to control his arms.

8-5: Use the basic defense to get one hand free, then immediately deliver a palm-heel strike to his nose or chin. That will get his attention! Or use your free hand to stab your finger tips at his eyes. He'll forget all about holding you the instant your dirty fingernails get near his baby blues. Of the five counterattacks in this group, this is the one I favor for actual use. Do not underestimate the life-saving value of simplicity.

ATTACK #9

The opponent grasps both of your wrists from behind.

38

BASIC DEFENSE #9

Unfortunately there is no simple wrist release to employ against an attacker who is holding your wrists from behind. You cannot simply twist against his thumbs because from behind your arms just don't twist in the right directions. This does not mean that you are helpless, however. It does mean that you will probably have to "resort to violence" to get free. If you are being assaulted this is not a problem, but against friends . . .

The two following counterattacks both begin with the same motion which you would do well to study.

Rotate your body a half-turn to your left, so that your left shoulder is toward the enemy. This motion wraps your right arm around behind your back as you turn. You will find in practice that you can easily grab his wrists during the turn.

Through this simple motion you have turned the tables on the opponent. Suddenly he realizes that the situation is no longer under his control. At this point you must be ready to break away if he releases you, or to counterattack if that is your decision. Personally, I recommend a sudden and violent counterattack in all situations where the opponent's intentions are evil rather than playful.

9-1: Perform the basic defense as described above, then lean to your right and use left side-thrust kicks to stomp on the opponent's shins, knees, thighs and groin. The knee is the best target if the situation is really serious. Note that your pulling hold on his arms will magnify the impact of your kick by denying him the ability to give way before the blow. Also, your hold on the opponent will help stabilize your balance, making it easier to kick repetitively without getting your foot back down on the ground. (See Figure 16.)

9-2: This one is a little harder but it works well once you get the knack. Start turning to the left as you twist your hands in his grip and tightly grasp his wrists. Continue to turn to your left, using your right hand to pull him forward behind your turning back. Plant your left leg outside of the opponent's right foot to trip him. Your continuing turn will pull him across your outstretched leg. He will fall heavily

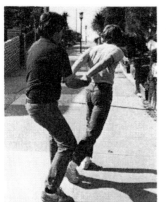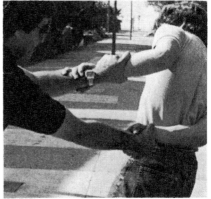

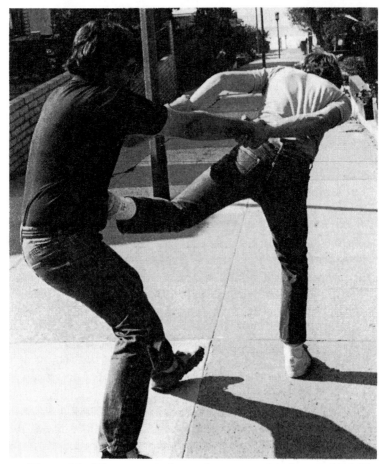

Figure 16: When an attacker grabs your wrists from behind it's hard to be clever about escaping. Usually a simple brute-force technique is the best bet here. Notice in these photos how the victim has turned the tables on the attacker by grasping the attacker's wrists before kicking.

on his right shoulder, possibly breaking his collarbone. This technique is best performed as a sudden spinning throw and requires either perfect timing or relatively great strength. Use it for demonstrations, but think twice about trying it in earnest unless it feels very natural to you.

9-3: Here's one for the more advanced students. This technique must begin with a stomp to the attacker's instep, to keep him from kicking too fast later on. Just glance down to find his right foot, lift your right knee to waist level, and then stamp down on the top of his foot about an inch in front of the shin. Think of it as if you were trying to stamp on a quart jar and break it. Now that you have his attention you can go on to the real counterattack.

Step slightly backward so your back brushes the attacker's chest. Then drop down on your knees (or into a crouch), bending your elbows and bringing your fists up in front of your shoulders. This motion will tear your wrists out of his grip. Twist immediately to the left and put your left forearm against his left knee, just below the kneecap. If you did any damage with your instep attack his weight will be on this leg and there will be no danger of getting kicked in the teeth; but keep your arm against his knee anyway. Then jerk his left heel out from under him with your right hand. As he falls, keep your left arm ready to deflect a possible kick from his right foot. Retreat and rise. (See Figure 17.)

Buried within the above technique is an extremely effective throw, the violence of which you will appreciate as soon as you try it in practice. The key is to hold his knee stationary while you jerk his heel forward. Most students mistakenly try to hold the foot in place while pushing on the knee, which doesn't work. I'll return to this throw in another technique where its utility will be even greater.

9-4: Turn to your left, swinging your right arm high up over your head as you turn. The attacker's forearm will pass above your head at the midpoint of the turn and he'll lose his grip on your right wrist at almost the same moment. As you are turning, twist your left hand in his grip to grasp his wrist, and then pull his left arm out straight. Your twisting

41

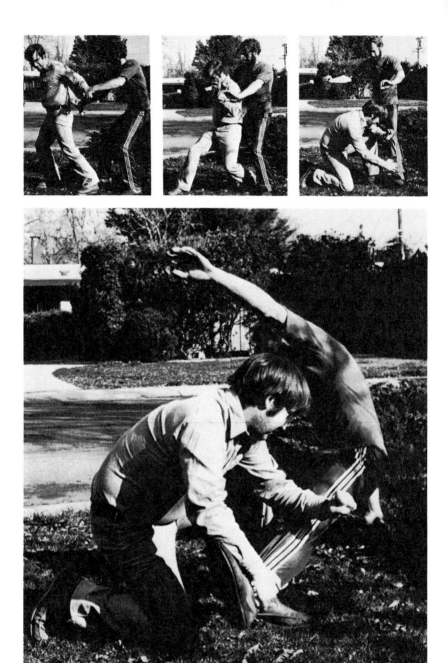

Figure 17: When someone you don't want to hospitalize grasps
your wrists from behind, you can free yourself by stepping straight
back and raising your hands to shoulder level. Then, if you wish, you
can drop on one knee and yank the jerk's leg out from under him. Notice in the third photo that the defender is on guard against a possible
kick as he drops into position for the throw.

motion will naturally rotate his arm to put the back of his elbow on top. Strike downward with your right fist to dislocate his elbow, or you can just apply a straight arm bar as in technique 4-1.

3. ESCAPES FROM CHOKES & LAPEL GRIPS

The neck and throat form a conduit which connects your brain to the rest of your body. Through this conduit pass the oxygen you must have to stay alive, the blood without which your brain will die within brief minutes, and the many incoming and outgoing nerve impulses which govern your entire existence. When someone grabs your throat he literally takes your life in his hands, and even if he is joking you may be only a fraction of a second from permanent—lethal—injury. There is no time to hesitate, no excuse for equivocation or delay. You must act decisively to free yourself and, if necessary, to render the attacker incapable of further violence.

Remember, when he has you by the throat it isn't a question of being humiliated or relieved of your credit cards. It's your life, your future years, which are on the line. Those future years will depend on your decisiveness, courage, and speed.

ATTACK #10

The attacker tries to choke you from in front, using both hands to squeeze your throat. He may place his thumbs on your trachea, or on the arteries beneath the corners of your jaw, or he may just squeeze in an unsophisticated manner.

If he crushes the trachea, which isn't difficult, you will strangle to death very unpleasantly as the windpipe swells shut, even if he releases you immediately. A few seconds of pressure on the carotid arteries will render you unconscious and helpless; a few minutes will leave you dead or brain-damaged. The untutored squeezer may not manage to accomplish either of these objectives, but his grip will be terribly painful.

I suggest that you avoid using your thumbs on your practice partner's neck while trying these moves. It is too easy to make mistakes. Just clasp him around the neck with your palms and fingers, keeping your thumbs free.

BASIC DEFENSE #10

By far the best immediate defense against a front choke is the forearm wedge. Of course a finger in the eye or a good swift kick aren't bad responses either, but the wedge works well, is very fast, and gives you the option of escape without injuring the opponent if he happens to be your brother-in-law the jerk.

The forearm wedge consists of clasping your hands (palms together) and spreading your elbows slightly to form a triangular wedge of your forearms. Start with your hands at about waist level and then drive your arms up between his forearms with great speed and force. Pretend to yourself that you're trying to strike an invisible target in the arc over your head. On the way the wedge formed by your forearms will lift and separate the attacker's hands away from your neck.

This technique is a favorite of mine for three reasons. First, it is a brute force move with no need for fancy timing. Anybody can learn to do it in minutes. Second, the rising wedge derives its power from the muscles of your back and shoulders (not your arms), which makes the motion fairly powerful even when performed by a 105-pound stewardess. Third, the forearm wedge takes advantage of your natural tendency to arch your back and pull away from a choke. I have found that the really successful self-defense techniques usually build on the student's first instinctive reaction to the attack. This one is a good example.

COUNTERATTACKS FOR SITUATION #10

10-1: Drive this wedge violently up between his forearms to tear his hands off your neck, then slam your clenched hands down into his face. This is the standard recommended technique in most of the military manuals and self-defense books, but in practice I have found it to be a little difficult to perform. Usually the opponent's face is just slightly out of reach, which forces you to lean forward awkwardly to deliver the blow. This robs the blow of its power.

I feel that the downward blow is best used when the opponent is pushing you backwards against a wall while he chokes you. In this case suddenly tearing his hands loose from your neck makes him lunge forward—directly into the path of your descending blow. If you can, use a hammer-fist blow (or its equivalent) against the bridge of his nose, and be satisfied if you can just rake your knuckles forcefully across his eyes, nose, and lips. A palm-heel strike up under his chin might be a good way to follow up. (See Figure 18.)

10-2: Here's one for the wrestlers among us. Use the forearm wedge as before, but separate your arms at the top of their rise, swing them out sideways and then back in to strike his lower ribs on each side. This is a simultaneous double hammer-fist attack. For extra power, strike downward at a 45-degree angle as if trying to bring your fists together at the level of his belt buckle. Finish by driving your shoulder into his abdomen as you encircle his thighs with your arms and pull up, throwing him on his back.

This technique has always seemed a little crude to me, since it depends on a wrestler's kind of strength and aggressiveness. This opens the question of who in his right mind would try to choke such a person, but then maybe the attacker isn't in his right mind. The key point to remember here is to avoid the tendency to bring the fists in horizontally toward his lower ribs. This weakens the blow. By angling the fists more downward as they hit the ribs you can add a lot more force to the attack.

10-3: This technique is one I learned from watching Bill Cosby do it on "I Spy" many years ago. It probably ought to remain in reserve for TV episodes where it would always work, but it is kind of fun and I'll pass it along to you.

Break the choke hold with the forearm wedge. At the

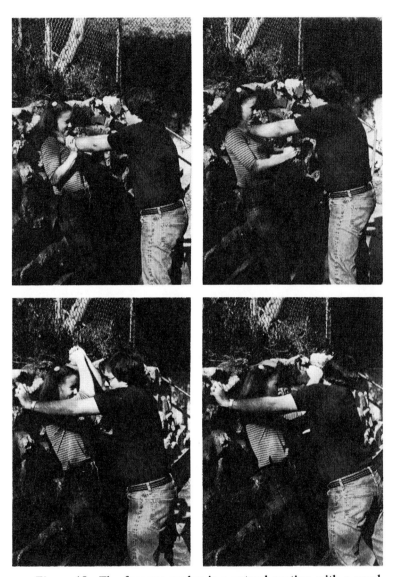

Figure 18: The forearm wedge is a natural motion with a good chance of success against a front choke. The follow-up blow to the face, however, works best when the attacker is pushing you against a wall or fence as shown here. He falls forward into the blow.

same time take a slight step forward. When your hands reach the top of their rise, separate them, swing them out and down, and then bring them together again at waist level. Performed correctly, this technique traps the opponent's wrists under your armpits. Now perform another forearm wedge . . . and dislocate both of his elbows at the same time!

10-4: Perform the basic defense as before. When you have knocked his hands free of your neck, reach out and grab his hipbones, then pull his pelvis toward you to meet your rapidly rising knee. Actually, this one will work just as well without the basic defense. When he grabs your neck, grab his hips and knee him hard in the genitals. He'll let go of your neck, do not doubt it.

10-5: Now for a simple throw. For some reason self-defense students (and their relatives) expect that the class will involve throwing people on the ground with bone-shattering results. I try to give them a little of what they expect now and then to keep them happy.

The first thing to understand about throws is that they require no strength. For novices this is very difficult to accept, but a properly timed, well-executed throw requires as little strength as punching someone backwards off a log. The principle is very much the same. All you do is set him up so he is tottering on the edge of an abyss, then you nudge him over. Of course, if the throw isn't timed right or the attempt is clumsy, strength begins to count a lot. In that case, the stronger you are the more likely it is that you will be able to salvage the situation and complete the throw, after a fashion.

Use the forearm wedge to break his hold. Bring your left hand down and grasp his right wrist. Step in toward him with your right foot, put your weight on it, and begin a continuing pivot to your left. As you turn catch his neck in the fold of your right elbow. Continue the pivot until your back is toward your opponent. It will work best if you squat down slightly so that your hips are lower than his.

This is the tricky part. Use your hold on his neck and arm to pull his shoulders *horizontally* around to your left, straightening your legs at the same time. Don't try to pull him forward or down. As you pull his head across your body and around to your left, his body will rock up and balance on your hip or lower back. When you practice this move experiment a little and search for this teeter-totter position. Once you have achieved this critical balance, only a slight additional pull will drop him on the ground in front of you. You see? Like falling off a log.

10-6: Here's another throw, which is far more subtle. Break the choke hold as before, then bring your hands down and grasp the opponent's shoulders or upper arms. Snap your right knee up into his groin to get his attention. (Actually the idea is to distract his attention.) Now shift the position of your right leg to put the knee against his left inguinal fold (the crease between his left upper thigh and his groin), while you slip your right heel around to the left spot behind his right knee. Once in position, it is a simple matter to spin him down to the ground by pushing with your knee, pulling with your heel and twisting his shoulders around to your left. (Pull with your left hand as you push with your right.) (See Figure 19.)

This trick sounds really esoteric until you try it and see for yourself how well it works. The hard part is getting into position. After that it's all downhill.

ATTACK #11

The two-handed front choke, just as in attack #10. It is the defense which differs.

BASIC DEFENSE #11

There is another basic defense for the front choke which works almost as well as the forearm wedge.

Clasp your hands over your head. In one forceful motion, step back with your left foot and twist your body to the left, catching his wrists under your right armpit. For additional power bow slightly from the waist as you twist. This motion rips his hands free of your neck or at least makes it very difficult for him to continue to throttle you.

This basic defense leaves you in a highly contorted, left-twisted stance at the moment your neck becomes free.

50

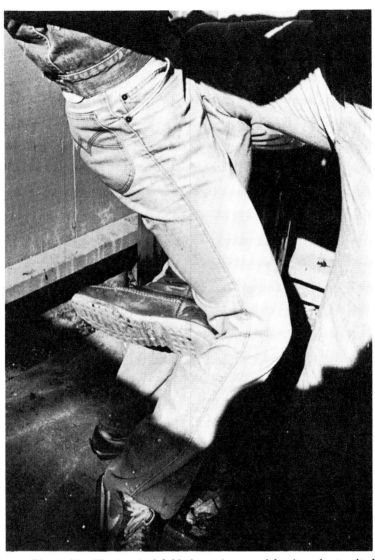

Figure 19: The inguinal fold throw is a specialty item best suited to relatively friendly scuffles . . . as you'll notice by the short distance from the opponent's knee to the defender's crotch.

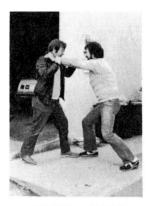 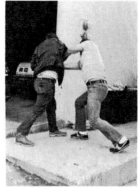 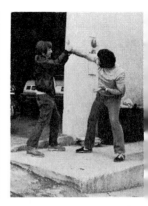

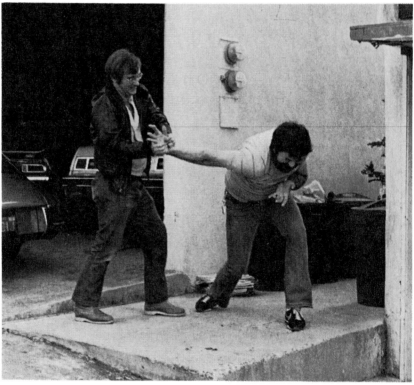

Figure 20: One excellent release from a front choke is to raise your right arm and twist violently to the left. Then, if you prefer, you can go on to a painful wristlock.

Counterattacks from this position tend to take advantage of the coil-recoil effect by using the body's natural tendency to whip back to the right from this position.

COUNTERATTACKS FOR SITUATION #11

11-1: Perform the basic defense as described above. If the attacker has been pulled off balance toward you (which can easily happen) snap your torso back to the right and catch him in the face with the back of your right elbow. This can be an extremely powerful blow, equivalent to striking him with a club.

11-2: The next technique incorporates a wristlock. Wristlocks are extremely useful little techniques which allow a small, unmuscular person to control and subdue a much larger assailant. This ability is usually of the greatest interest to police officers, but occasionally the rest of us discover a need to immobilize someone without breaking his leg or knocking him out. Wristlocks are the key to this kind of control.

Use the basic defense to free your throat, but make an effort to trap his wrists by clamping them under your right arm as you turn. To perform this technique you need to keep at least a minimum amount of control over his hands during the twisting stage. At the completion of the leftward twist, when your neck is free, take his right hand in your hands.

Pay close attention because this works only one way. Your right hand should grasp the little-finger side of the attacker's palm. Your fingers will be in his palm and your thumb will be on the back of his hand near the knuckle of his middle finger. Your left hand grasps the thumb side of his hand, with your fingers in his palm and your thumb on the back of his hand near the knuckle of his middle finger. (Some military manuals show the thumbs crossed in an "X" but this is not necessary.)

Now you have him. Keeping your hands in close to your chest, twist your body back around to the right until you are facing him again. Keep his hand turned so that his finger tips point up. To apply pressure against his wrist joint, simply

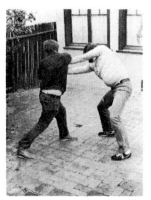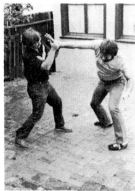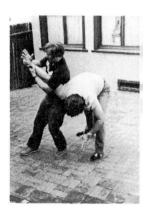
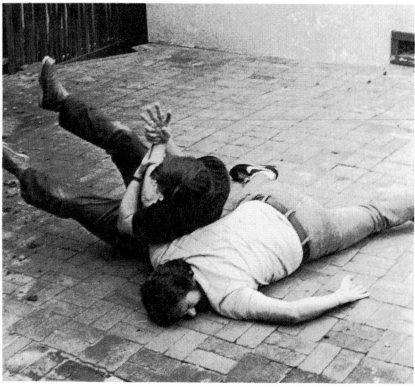

Figure 21: Another response to the front choke is to break the hold as in Figure 20, and then use the wristlock to set up this very brutal takedown. Once you have captured the opponent's arm (third photo) all you have to do is lean back and throw your feet out to drive his head into the bricks.

pull his arm toward you with your fingers while pressing the other way with your thumbs. The pain is very sharp and impossible to ignore. By applying pain with the wristlock and simultaneously twisting his hand to your right, you can make him bend over at the waist and beg for mercy. If you feel no such emotion, a swift kick in the teeth will take the fight out of him. (See Figure 20.)

11-3: If the finesse of a wristlock seems a little feminine to you, here's a good, crude, brute-force variation which the male macho types can sink their teeth into. Twist free and grab his right hand as described in the previous technique. Turn back to your right, twisting his arm to keep his finger tips pointing up. This will result in rotating the back of his elbow upward, too.

Let go with your left hand, retaining your grip with your right hand. Pivot to the right on your right foot and catch his captured arm under your left armpit. Try to catch his arm just below the shoulder. Put your left hand under his wrist, maintaining your grip with your right hand.

At this point you can exert pressure against his wrist by pulling with your right hand. You can put painful pressure on his elbow joint by levering upward on his wrist with your left hand (the right hand helps, too). But most people prefer the final option. Lever up on his wrist with both hands as you throw your feet out from under you and let your entire weight hang on his upper arm. (The motion is like sitting down on the ground very suddenly.) Unless your opponent has superhuman strength and resistance to pain, he'll crash headfirst to the pavement. He'll think he was hit by a passing truck just as he was about to choke the life out of you. (See Figure 21.)

11-4: A very simple counterattack which derives from basic defense #11 consists of breaking the hold by spinning to the left (as always), but then you continue the spin and perform a complete 360-degree turn. As you are coming around stick out your left elbow and hit him in the face or ribs, as appropriate. A hammer-fist attack can also be of use here under some circumstances.

55

ATTACK #12

The two-handed front choke, just as before.

BASIC DEFENSE #12

There is one more choke escape which I want to tell you about because it is very elegant—and it also works quite well. It appeals to nonviolent types more than to the machos, but then again, "self-defense isn't just for jocks anymore."

The attacker has both hands on your neck choking you. Place your hands together in front of your chest in an attitude of prayer. Raise your hands to a point between his wrists. Bow forward slightly and place your chin between the tips of your fingers. As you continue to bow forward, slide your hands up along either side of the edge of your jaw, under your ears, until they meet again behind your neck. Bow low, turn to one side, and step away. You're free. (See Figure 22.)

I really ought to point out to inexperienced readers that you are very vulnerable to a knee in the face during the bow, so make it fast if you can. You can't bow faster than he can kick, but you can bow faster than he can think of kicking, which is just as good.

I offer no counterattacks to go with this escape, because it just wouldn't be in keeping with the humble spirit of the technique. One simply bows in deep respect and steps away. Of course one simultaneously makes the attacker look like a total fool, but there is no need to be arrogant about it, is there?

ATTACK #13

At this point we shift from front chokes to lapel grips. A *lapel grip* is that classic TV confrontation where the bad guy grabs you by the shirt front and snarls, "Smile when you say that." Okay, now you can smile and simultaneously make him wish he had never laid eyes on you.

BASIC DEFENSE #13

The following two counterattacks serve as their own basic defenses, but both require that you keep your cool

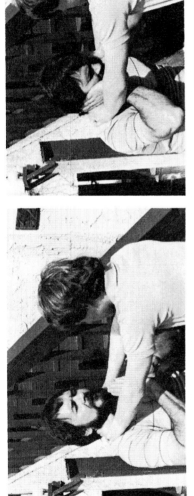

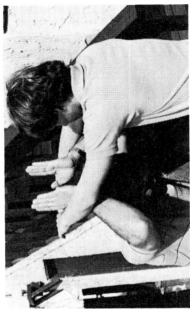

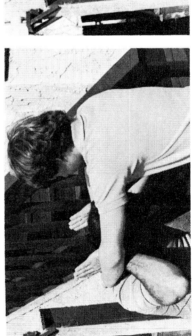

Figure 22: It might happen that your kid brother grabs your neck and won't let go, but killing or castrating him would distress the family. This non-violent Aikido technique will free you without injuring anyone.

57

and stay on guard to parry that ominous right fist the adversary is certainly shaking in your face. Also, when you see that he is reaching for your shirt, you must naturally and smoothly bring your hands up on either side of his wrist. If you do this as an immediate reaction he won't really notice it, but if you wait too long and then reach for his arm he'll know that something is up.

Therefore, in this case your basic defense is simply to get your hands on the fist that is tearing your shirt.

COUNTERATTACKS FOR SITUATION #13

13-1: The attacker grasps your lapel with his left fist, thumb up, and threatens to punch you with his right fist. (You'll be able to feel the position of his fist with your hands. If the palm of his fist is facing up, not the thumb, use the next technique instead.)

Pass your left hand over the top of his fist, curling your fingers around the little-finger edge of his hand. Use your grip to twist his fist to your left (counterclockwise) so that the back of his fist is uppermost. Clamp his fist securely against your chest with your left hand, forcing his wrist to bend enough to get the heel of his fist pressed tightly against your chest. Turning slightly to the left, raise your right elbow over the attacker's arm and then smash it down against the back of his forearm just behind the wrist.

The leverage of this motion is so extreme that you may be able to snap the bones of his arm like a pair of matchsticks. Note that there is a scissoring motion implied here. The back of your upper arm and the lateral edge of your chest form the blades of the scissors. As you bring your elbow down his arm gets "cut" between them.

A milder application of this hold will bend the forearm bones, which is just as painful as it sounds. He'll drop instantly on his knees to relieve the pressure. At that point you can casually snap your right fist out in a reverse hammer blow to the face. Of course, the really appropriate thing to do is to force him to kneel and then say, "On your knees, dog, when you speak to your betters." (See Figure 23.)

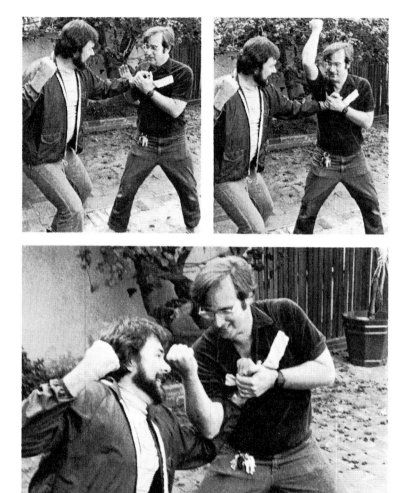

Figure 23: When someone threatens you by grabbing the front of your shirt you can trap his fist and snap the bones in his forearm quite handily. If he makes any threatening moves with that upraised fist do a hammer-fist attack to his face instead.

At any point you may defend against a right-hand punch by blocking with the left hand, or, when the hold is applied by delivering a pre-emptive hammer strike to the face.

13-2: This technique is for those times when the attacker's grip on your collar leaves his fist with the palm up. In this case you can't establish the proper hold for technique 13-1, but never fear. There is an equally effective alternative.

Grasp his fist with both hands, curling you fingers around into his palm and putting you thumbs on the back of his hand near the middle knuckle. (Do you recognize the wrist-lock again?)

Take a step back to pull his arm out straight. Apply pressure against the wrist joint by bending his fist toward the inside of his forearm. He won't be able to maintain his grip on your shirt. To drop him on his back, pull his hand toward your hip as you twist his arm sharply to your right. To relieve the pain in his wrist and arm he'll obligingly flop right over on his back. If you are not feeling charitable, your next move is to wafflestomp his face with the sole of your hiking boot. If you *are* feeling charitable, perhaps a kick in the ear would be sufficient.

4. ESCAPES FROM HEADLOCKS

A very common event in a barnyard-type fight is for one of the opponents to catch the other in some kind of headlock. You see this especially among kids and a few men who haven't learned anything about fighting since they were in grade school. It is also very prevalent on TV wrestling shows. Although headlocks look very effective to a novice, when one of these bovine bullies puts a headlock on a knowledgeable self-defense student he places his dignity, and his life itself, in deadly peril. It should go without saying that self-defense students are advised to avoid the use of headlocks under most circumstances. The only exceptions are those locks which result in instant unconsciousness or death, and therefore offer little opportunity for retaliation.

ATTACK #14

Attack #14 is a classic under-the-arm headlock, in which *your opponent has clamped your head under his right arm.* In this position you are both facing the same direction, your left ear is against his body and your left shoulder is against his right kidney. Notice that his left hand is free and may be used to strike you in the face. Both of your hands are free. The retaliatory potential of this situation is enormous. So is the danger.

BASIC DEFENSE #14

In this case the fundamental defense is extremely simple. The key is to immobilize his left arm so he can't hit you with

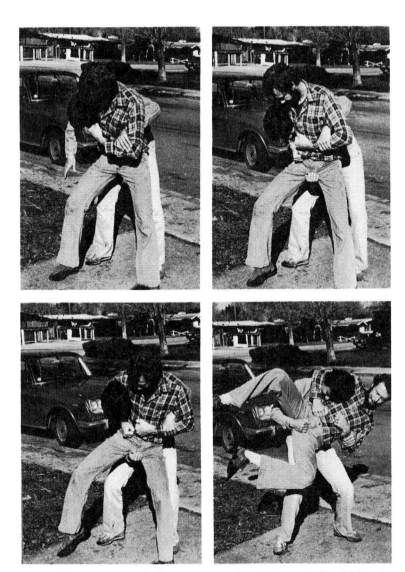

Figure 24: A headlock is a common but ludicrous hold which puts the attacker at a severe disadvantage. First you have to pin the attacker's left arm to protect your face from punches. Then grab his private parts and pick him up by them! You can easily turn him upside down and drop him on his head with this technique. It doesn't take as much strength as you might think.

it. After his left arm is neutralized you can take your time and pick one of several effective counterattacks.

To immobilize the attacker's left arm, just reach around his back with your left arm and insert your hand between his chest and upper arm. Turn your palm outward and grasp his bicep just above the elbow. You'll find that he'll have a hard time breaking loose from this simple hold. While he is trying, he won't notice the beginning of your counterattack until too late.

COUNTERATTACKS FOR SITUATION #14

14-1: If the attacker has tried to punch you in the face use the basic defense described above to neutralize his left arm, otherwise use your left hand to reach up over his right shoulder and get your fingernails into his eyes. This will force his head up and back while simultaneously distracting him from all other thoughts other than getting his eyes away from your fingers.

Use your right hand to reach between his legs from behind and firmly grasp his genitals. (He will be having sudden second thoughts about the fight at this point.) Straighten up, lifting him by the genitals and driving his face backward and down with your left hand. His body will rock backwards over your left hip like a teeter-totter. All you have to do is raise his feet up high and then fall backwards to bring his skull into violent contact with the pavement.

If your left hand is busy immobilizing his arm just grab his genitals and forget about clawing at his eyes. It isn't as easy to throw him without a hand on his face but it can still be done. Try it and see. (See Figure 24.)

14-2: A variation of the above technique is to hook your right arm under his right knee, catching the leg in the crook of your elbow. (Do not grasp his leg with your hand!) If you straighten up he'll rock back across your left hip as before, and if you are fairly strong you will be able to lift him right up in the air (the leverage is tremendous). At this point you'll be holding him horizontally across your chest, belly up, with his feet about as high as his head. To bring the situation to a sudden and permanent end, kneel suddenly and let him drop across your bent left knee. Drop him so that your knee catches him just above the base of the spine— breaking his back. Even if his back isn't broken the whiplash of his fall will slam his head into the ground very forcefully. He might not survive it.

14-3: What if you just can't lift him? Some women and frail men are so convinced of their weakness that they just won't give a throw a decent try. I think it is important to give people alternative techniques they can believe in, even if the problem is really in their minds. Therefore, here is a throw which does not require any dramatic lifting.

Put the sole of your left foot against the back of the opponent's left heel. Claw at his eyes with your left hand and hook your right arm under his right knee as before. Use your attack on his eyes and your hold on his leg to encourage him to lose his balance to the rear. He'll try to recover by hopping back on his left leg, but your foot prevents this. He'll fall heavily to the rear.

14-4: It is possible that the opponent may release you as he falls. This is pretty common and it is to be hoped for. If not, you will almost certainly wind up on top and then have to continue the fight from the gorund.

The preceding techniques tend to leave the attacker lying on his left side, with you poised over him on your hands and knees. We assume that he still has your neck encircled with his right arm. Otherwise you would have escaped by now.

To get free, grab his hair or gouge his eyes with your left hand, driving his head back and forcing him to arch his back. Once you have him distracted, grasp his right wrist with your right hand and start backing up with your knees, pulling your head and his arm back behind him to the point where your head slips free and you have him in an arm lock. This technique works well because you can use the strength of your legs and torso against his unassisted right arm. (See Figure 25.)

Note that if he holds his right hand with his left, you will not be able to pull his arm back until you gouge his eyes. If he is human he'll use his left hand to protect his eyes and you

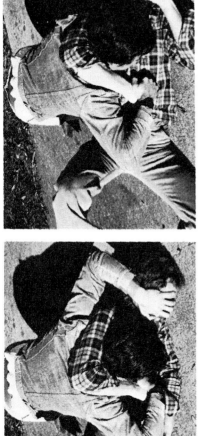

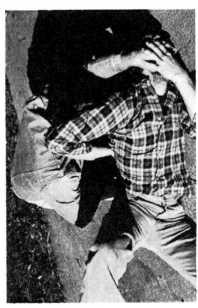

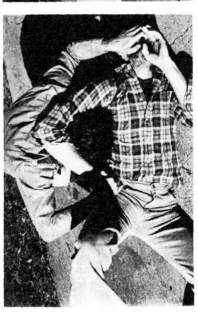

Figure 25: What if the attacker doesn't let go of your head when you throw him on the ground (Figure 24)? Claw at his eyes to make him arch his back, and then crawl straight backward until you have him in a hammer lock.

65

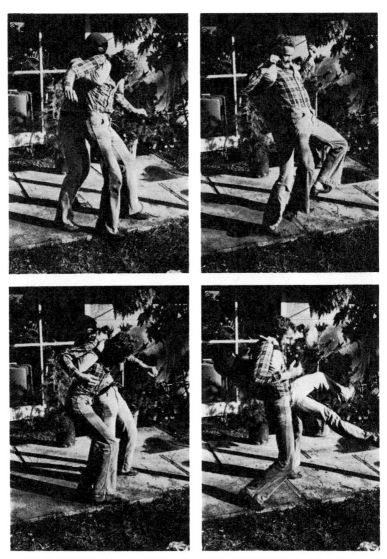

Figure 26: The standing full nelson is a common hold that is both dangerous and difficult to escape from. The escape begins by stomping on both of the attacker's insteps at once. Then step around to get your leg behind him and throw him on his back.

can proceed with the escape. Another little trick which can be useful here is a snappy knee kick into his kidney. A couple of these kicks will certainly give him second thoughts about continuing to hold your head.

14-5: If you still can't get loose, or if you fouled up and the bad guy is on top after the throw, simply start using elbows, knees, teeth, fingers, and fists as viciously as you know how. This is supposed to be dirty fighting, not a wrestling match. No one will disqualify you for doing unmentionable things to the opponent's kidneys, solar plexus, groin, eyes, throat, and ribs. Force him to let go of your head just to defend himself. You will find that it is a very effective technique.

ATTACK #15

The attacker has placed you in a full nelson hold from behind, and is using the strength of his arms and the weight of his body in an attempt to break your neck. In a full nelson hold the attacker stands behind you, slips his arms under yours, and then laces his fingers together behind your neck. In this position he can exert severe pressure against your cervical vertebrae. It is vital that you relieve this pressure immediately.

BASIC DEFENSE #15

This situation is a little different from the others in this book in that the basic defense technique can only be applied after one of the counterattacks. In the previous techniques the basic defense has opened the way to a selection of responses. This time, however, the various responses all lead to the same ending position and final release.

A defense against a full nelson requires that you relieve the pressure on your neck. The only unfailing way to do this is to drop the attacker flat on his back and land on top of him. In this position he cannot exert maximum pressure against your neck because he can't use his weight against you.

At that point you can break the hold easily by reaching

behind your neck and prying up one of his fingers. Bend it backwards until it snaps. He'll let go.

A word of caution. Don't try to reach for his fingers before dropping him on his back or you will make your situation worse instead of better. Reaching up behind your neck while still standing raises your elbows and lets him consolidate his hold. Remember: until you have him on his back you must keep your elbows pulled down tightly against your sides. It is the only thing you can do to interfere with his leverage against your neck.

COUNTERATTACKS FOR SITUATION #15

15-1: Try a back snap kick to the groin or a stomp on the instep to get his attention and distract him from pressing on your neck. A back snap kick consists of snapping your heel up behind you as if to hit yourself in the hip pocket, only you make sure that his groin is in the way. If you happen to hit his shin or kneecap instead, the distraction will still be sufficient to increase the probability of overall success.

Step back between his legs with your right foot. Throw your weight back into his left shoulder, and as his balance shifts to the left, use your right foot to hook his right leg and swing it forward and up as far as possible. Let your weight shift to the right and brace yourself for a jolt. He'll fall like a felled tree and you'll land on top. If you can, land hard. (See Figure 26.)

It may be that the shock of the fall will be sufficient to free you, in which case your momentum will naturally lead to a backward somersault out of the hold. If not, resort to the basic defense to break one of his fingers and force him to release you.

Please be cautious when practicing this technique. You could hospitalize your practice partner very easily by dropping on him too hard by mistake, and there is some potential for injury to your neck, too. Practice partners sometimes hang on tighter than real opponents because they know what is coming and can't be surprised. In this case it can be dangerous.

15-2: Keep your elbows clamped down tightly against

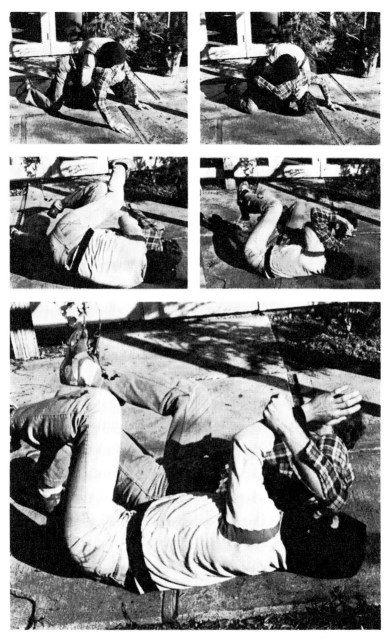

Figure 27: If the technique shown in Figure 26 doesn't quite get you free you may wind up in this unenviable position, on all fours with the neck hold still in place. To escape, clamp his right arm under yours and do a shoulder roll. With the attacker on the bottom you can reach back and break one of his fingers to get free. An elbow to the face is a good parting gesture.

your sides to keep him from getting too much leverage against your neck. Start the festivities by suddenly picking up both feet and stamping your heels hard on the tops of his feet just in front of the shins. He'll be stunned and immobilized. Leap to the right and swing your left leg around behind him. Plant your left foot behind and between his feet.

You are now in a position in which you can rock the opponent backward across your left hip just by straightening up and shoving back with your left shoulder against his chest. To drop him on his back drive your hips forward into him as you smash your left elbow back into his face. He'll fall heavily, but you'll land on top. Use the basic defense to break the hold and roll away.

15-3: It is possible that you may find yourself subjected to a full nelson hold while on your hands and knees. For one thing, one of the previous two throws may go slightly wrong, ending with you on all fours and your opponent kneeling over you with the neck-breaking hold still intact. (For the sake of discussion, we'll assume that your opponent is kneeling on your left side.)

The basic idea is the same as before. You must get your opponent on his back before you can break the hold. To do this, lift your right hand and grasp his right forearm. Clamp his arm tightly between your arm and chest. Now roll forward and to your right, tucking in your right shoulder. Your attacker will be irresistibly drawn over your back and rolled onto the floor. The ending position leaves him on his back with you on top. Wrench one of his fingers out of its socket and roll free. (See Figure 27.)

5. DEFENSE FROM THE GROUND

It is easy to imagine a situation in which you have been knocked off your feet but your opponent is still upright. It is therefore very important that you understand how to fight from the ground against a standing opponent, and especially important to know how and when to try to get up again. If you try to rise prematurely you'll get kicked in the ribs, teeth, or groin every time.

I think you'll find this section to be somewhat unusual. I have never seen the techniques of supine fighting against a standing attacker expressed in a book, and it may be that this is the only treatment of the subject in print. This is difficult to understand because these are among the most effective and reliable techniques in the self-defense field. They are devastating against even a highly trained fistfighter, and they leave a knifeman feeling helpless and distraught. Obviously this section is well worth your close attention.

ATTACK #16

This could be one of several situations in which *you have wound up on your back while a single opponent stands threateningly over you.* Maybe you were knocked down, or maybe you dropped onto your back deliberately. The latter course would be wise if the attacker is brandishing a knife or club, or if he has shown signs of having significant skill with his fists.

BASIC DEFENSE #16

The first rule of fighting from the ground is never to get up while your opponent is capable of kicking or striking you.

71

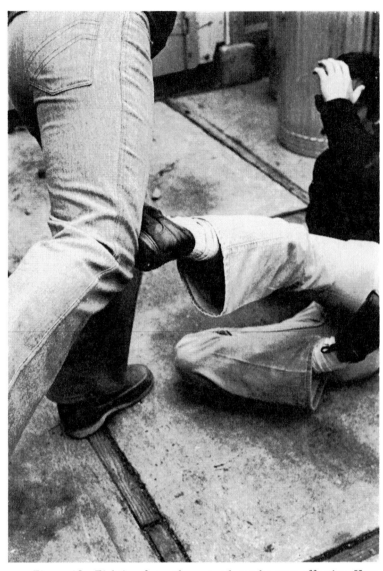

Figure 28: Fighting from the ground can be very effective. Here
the defender catches a would-be kicker in the knee . . . a very painful
and disruptive block. Notice that the defender is using his other foot to
cover his groin in case the kick gets by.

Curl up with your knees raised in front of your chest, your elbows tight in against your sides and your hands held above your chest in front of your face. Stay on your back, using your hands and elbows to pivot your body around on the base of your spine, keeping your feet directed toward the opponent.

You may find that you will have to use one of your feet now and then to assist in spinning your body around as the attacker desperately tries to outmaneuver you and get past the guard of your feet and legs. Just be sure that you keep at least one foot cocked and ready to kick at all times. Two is better.

This defensive position is nearly impregnable once you have given it a little practice. Nearly everyone can spin around on his back much faster than an attacker can run in a circle around him. This forces him to attack you over your legs, which are not only immensely strong but also partially armored. Think about trying to stick a knife blade through the sole of your shoe and you'll see what I mean.

Remember to keep your shins up high enough to block any attempted kick to your abdomen, but also low enough to protect your groin, too. It isn't hard to do this, but you do have to think about it. Your hands serve as a second line of defense ready to catch or deflect a kick or an object thrown at your head.

You can test the efficacy of this defense in practice by taking the position and then asking your partner to try to touch your head with his hand. Make a lively contest of it and you will soon see that no matter what direction he dodges you will be able to keep up with him. He will always find your ready feet between him and his goal.

COUNTERATTACKS FOR SITUATION #16

16-1: The most obvious counterattack is actually an integral part of the basic defense itself. Kick the bastard! Every time he comes close lash out with a foot and kick him in the knee, shin, groin, and even in the hands if he reaches out for you. Don't be hesitant about it. Kick fast and viciously, and don't stop until he is obviously hurt. As usual, the knees are the best target. (See Figure 28.)

16-2: You can carry the attack to the opponent by rising up crab-style on your palms and heels and scuttling toward him, lashing out with your feet at his shins. I know this doesn't sound like what your favorite TV hero would do, but when the bad guys aren't getting paid to fall down it's nice to have a tactic that is both effective and unusual. You'll be amazed to see how wildly your practice partner has to dance and scramble to keep out of your way. The effect on an actual attacker is to demoralize him very quickly and, incidentally, to make him look foolish in front of spectators. Bullies can't stand being laughed at.

16-3: If you don't actually injure him with one of your kicks (which you may well do) you will certainly enrage him to the point of recklessness. He'll try to jump you . . . and he'll sing soprano for life.

You will have plenty of time. He'll brace himself, set his face in a mask of rage, give a big yell, take a running jump and come in at your face heels first. Don't worry, your hands can bat his feet far enough to the side to protect your head. Concentrate instead on positioning your foot in the path of his descending groin. Lock your knee and brace for the shock. He'll feel like he jumped out of the back of a pickup truck and accidentally straddled the top of a fence post on the way down. No matter, choirs need men with high voices.

If your opponent happens to be the reckless type who dives over your legs headfirst, you will have an opportunity to kill him with a kick to the throat. Failing that, your kick to the face, chest, collarbone, or abdomen will surely destroy his interest in continued combat.

16-4: A brighter than average opponent may try to kick you instead of attacking you with his hands. He may even try to kick your calf muscles to cramp them and cripple your defense. Your response to this tactic is to roll slightly to one side and use a side-thrust kick against his incoming shin.

This means that you wait until he cocks his legs for the kick, and then you intercept it by thrusting the outer edge of the sole of your shoe at his shin. Hold your foot horizontally to maximize your chances of intercepting his swinging leg. From his end it will feel like slamming his shin into the edge of a coffee table. One application of this block and he'll abruptly stop trying to kick you.

16-5: The next two techniques are takedowns, or throws, with which you can drop your opponent flat on the floor even though you are lying on your back and he is standing up. The throws work best if you have already succeeded in hurting him with a couple of shin and knee kicks, but if executed skillfully they will bring even an uninjured opponent into sudden and violent contact with the floor.

Assume that your opponent turns his right side toward you as he approaches, presenting the outside of his right leg to you. Roll on to your right hip and hook the top of his right foot (at the point where it meets the shin) with the back of your right heel. Use the top of your left foot to kick hard into the back of his knee. This will fold his leg. Roll violently a complete turn to your right, maintaining your holds on his knee and ankle as you roll. The combined effect is to buckle his leg and bend his ankle up behind his thigh. He'll either fall flat on his face or he'll drop heavily on his kneecap, either of which would be a welcome development.

This throw is best performed in a single, snappy rolling motion which rolls up the opponent's leg and also propels him forward off balance into the fall. If he lands on his belly and you still have his leg under control, this identical hold can be used to subdue him. Use your right ankle to keep the pressure on, forcing his heel down toward the back of his thigh. Since your other foot is caught in the fold of his knee, this pressure produces a nutcracker effect where your left ankle is the nut. In this case, however, the nut is far harder and bonier than the cracker. He'll yell for mercy. (See Figure 29.)

Of course this technique, like many others in this book, can also be used on the other side of the body. If he presents you with the side of his left leg you can just roll to the left and proceed from there.

16-6: There is another throw which works even better

than the last one. It is used when the opponent steps in directly toward you, not when he is facing to the side as before.

Assume that he has taken a step toward you with his left foot. Roll to the right and hook the top of your right foot around behind his left heel. Use your left foot to push firmly against his knee as you yank his heel toward you. This will drop him right on his butt with considerable force. He may not land on his back, but he'll be off his feet and badly shaken for several seconds.

Check back to technique 9-3 where this throw is performed using your hands instead of your feet.

16-7: Only after you have injured the attacker or dropped him on the ground can you attempt to get up again. This is essential. Unless you want him to go through the inconvenience of picking your teeth out of his shoelaces, you'd better hurt him enough to make him keep his distance before you rise.

When the time is right, turn your body so that your feet are pointed toward the attacker and then cautiously roll over on your hands and knees. Keep a weather eye out over your shoulder, and keep one foot cocked for a kick in case he tries to jump you. If the opponent does attack at this critical instant just lash out at his legs with your foot and roll over on your back again. Continue fighting on your back as before. Otherwise you may continue to rise. At this point I would strongly suggest a discreet retreat.

16-8: Another method of getting up is to half-face toward your wounded adversary as you sit up and carefully rise to your feet. Make sure that you are out of his reach, though. If he tries to rush you simply roll backward on to your back and fight as before.

ATTACK #17

The techniques examined so far for fighting from the ground are not effective in two specific situations. The first is when *you are fighting more than one person,* and cannot possibly keep both at bay at the same time. The other situa-

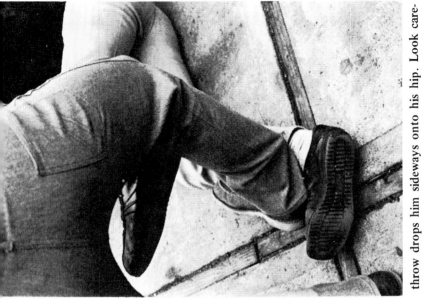

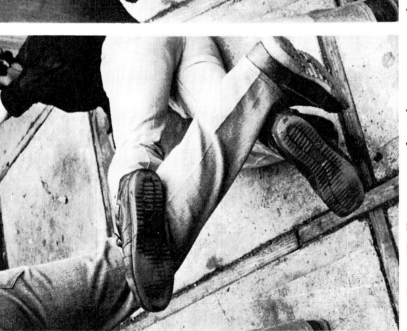

throw drops him sideways onto his hip. Look carefully at what the second throw does to the man's knee and ankle. Either throw may do enough damage to put the attacker down permanently.

Figure 29: Here are two foot throws to use against a standing opponent. The first spills the attacker forward onto his kneecap, while the second

tion is when *your opponent is too close to kick,* i.e., when he is sitting on your chest.

Suppose you get knocked down in a fight with two opponents. You can keep your feet toward one of them but the other is perfectly free to circle around and attack from the side or rear.

BASIC DEFENSE #17

First of all, if you are fighting more than one opponent you must not fall. Once on the ground you will certainly be kicked into submission unless you can roll and immediately spring back on to your feet. This kind of tumbling becomes second nature to judo students (and to the better karate students) but self-defense people usually don't have the time or the agility to spare on it. If possible, it is a skill well worth cultivating. Speed is your salvation in this situation.

If they close in on you too quickly for you to regain your feet, try to protect your vital organs by lying on your back. Clasp your hands behind your neck, tuck your head down, pull your knees up to your chin, and cross your ankles over your genitals. Rock your body around wildly as they kick you in an attempt to spoil their aim. An absolutely essential point is to yell and scream as if in great pain. Not only will this summon aid, but your attackers may decide that they have punished you enough and quit before actually injuring you seriously.

Obviously this is a last-ditch defense, only to be used in desperation. In this situation your chances of "winning" are minimal, and your application of self-defense concentrates mostly on limiting the amount of damage the attackers can do to you. If you get the chance, however, don't hesitate to lash out with a foot and dislocate somebody's knee. If you can work the odds down to one-on-one you can go on the offensive and emerge victorious.

ATTACK #18

This is that familiar playground situation in which you have been knocked on your back and *the attacker is trying to hold you down by sitting on your chest.* Although this hold-down is crude and unsophisticated, it is also very common. The utility of this hold-down in an attempted rape is too obvious to require comment.

For the purposes of discussion, we'll assume that the attacker may be trying to choke you with his hands as well as simply hold you down. If he is choking you, your response must be immediate. On the other hand, if he is just trying to hold you down you may have additional time to get your wits together and launch a more coordinated counter-offensive.

BASIC DEFENSE #18

In this case the basic defense is extremely simple. There will be a moment, perhaps as much as two or three seconds, during which the attacker will be busy trying to grab your arms and get on top of you. You should have ample opportunity to cock your leg and reposition his nose back between his ears. The kick could as easily be directed into his ribs, abdomen, or groin, and don't overlook a good solid stomp into the center of his thigh. In other words, the best defense is a pre-emptive kick wherever it will do the most good. Two or three of these will make him lose all interest in holding on to you.

If for some reason you can't employ this defense (maybe you're being tickled instead of raped) you'll have to rely on one of the following escapes or counterattacks. But be advised. None of them works quite as well as that boot heel in the eye.

COUNTERATTACKS FOR SITUATION #18

18-1: You are lying flat on your back and the attacker is straddling your abdomen, possibly intent on rape (if your gender is appropriate, or even if it isn't!). Draw your knees up until they touch his back, then dig in your heels, arch your back, and thrust yourself violently along the floor in the direction your head is pointing (out from under him). You may not make much progress on the first try so be ready to repeat the effort over and over as rapidly as you can. You'll find with a little practice that you can scoot yourself along on your back considerably faster than he can stump after you on his knees.

It will be an awkward contest, but at some point you'll get far enough ahead to get a foot free. At that point, without even a split second of hesitation, you must place the ball of your foot on his abdomen and viciously rip the soul of your shoe down his belly, between his legs, and out behind him. His heart and mind will follow.

18-2: This technique is a little less destructive than the last one. Pull your knees up as far as you can while keeping your feet flat on the floor. Plant your left foot firmly and let your right leg extend slightly. At the critical moment, use your left foot to heave your body off the ground, arching your back to lift and tilt the attacker forward. At the top of his rise slam your right thigh as hard as you can into his butt. It will also be helpful if you can strike him up under the armpits with your hands at the same instant.

The net effect is to catapult the opponent over your head (and slightly to your left). A naive, surprised enemy can find himself thrown a good eight or ten feet by this technique. I've seen it happen. Usually, though, you'll be doing well to knock him off at all. If you do succeed in spilling him to your left don't miss the opportunity to get in a kick or two. If you have time scramble to your feet and run.

18-3: The attacker is sitting on your chest choking you. Grasp the hair at the back of his head with your left hand (so that he cannot pull away). Then drive your right thumb into his left eye, pressing the thumb toward your left hand. He will try to pull his head away from the thumb. By pulling his hair to the left as your thumb explores his eye socket you can roll him off your chest. You'll find that this technique works even better if you use your thumbnail instead of the ball of your thumb.

18-4: Break the choke with a forearm wedge (basic defense #10). It works almost as well when you are lying down as well as standing up. Then grab his head (hair, ears, neck, shoulders, collar, or lapels) and yank his face down as you tuck in your chin and drive your bony forehead up to meet him. Sure, you'll cut your forehead, but a couple of stitches will fix you right up. The guy on top, however, is going to have some difficulty adjusting to his missing teeth, cut lips, and broken nose. Smack him in the face again just for luck, being sure to take the blow in the center of your forehead, and if he hasn't gotten the idea by then stick your thumb in his eye and roll him off as described in the previous technique.

18-5: This one is very satisfying because of its stunning speed. The attacker is sitting on your chest and choking you with both hands. Cross your wrists in front of your face and break the hold by pushing his hands out sideways from your neck. This requires a pair of snappy palm-heel strikes against the inside of his wrists. Note that this is not a slapping motion, but a short, sharp thrust with the heel of the hand. Do it with conviction and his hands will rip off your neck with no difficulty.

At this point your neck is free and your arms are crossed above your chest. The opponent's face is about two feet away, but is descending in response to having his arms knocked out of position. Uncross your forearms suddenly in a scissoring motion (one forearm sliding along the other like a pair of scissors blades) until your fists come to a jarring halt on opposite sides of his neck. For added power make the strike by spreading your elbows apart rather than by lashing out with your hands.

This strike to the neck can be made even more damaging by using a double knife-hand strike (chop) instead of your fists. The fist strike jars the nerves of the neck (see **Black Medicine Volume I**) but the knife-hand attack also injures the organs of the throat. Envision the knife-edge of your right hand smearing the top half of the opponent's larynx to the right, while your left hand in a scissoring motion drives the bottom half of his larynx violently to the left. The resulting anatomical shearing of the fellow's windpipe and vocal cords is left as an exercise for the reader's imagination.

81

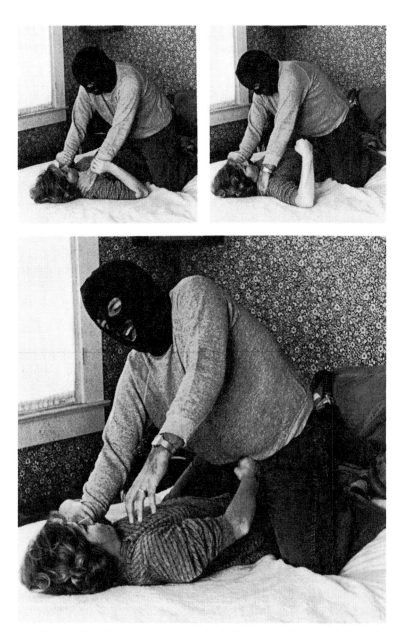

Figure 30: People tend to overlook the most obvious solutions to simple problems. Here no elaborate escape is necessary because the attacker's groin is within easy reach of the victim's fist!

If you take advantage of the coil-recoil motion implied here you can execute the whole technique, choke release and neck strike, in about half of one second. He'll never see it coming.

18-6: The attacker is sitting on your chest choking you as before, except that in the rictus of his frenzy he has hunched his shoulders and straightened his arms until the elbows locked. If you can see that his arms are held unnaturally straight, you can break the choke hold by clapping your hands sharply on the backs of his elbows. Hammer-fist blows work even better.

18-7: This technique is especially elegant, simple, unexpected, and effective. Use a fist blow or a palm-heel attack to his groin. It's right there within reach and he's not thinking about defending it. One lightning blow will take his mind off worldly affairs for a long time. (See Figure 30.)

18-8: Since your legs are free, you might as well see if you can use them. If you are limber you can pick up your right foot and dent his skull with the back of your heel. Try it and experiment a little to see what you can do. Remember, he'll never see it coming.

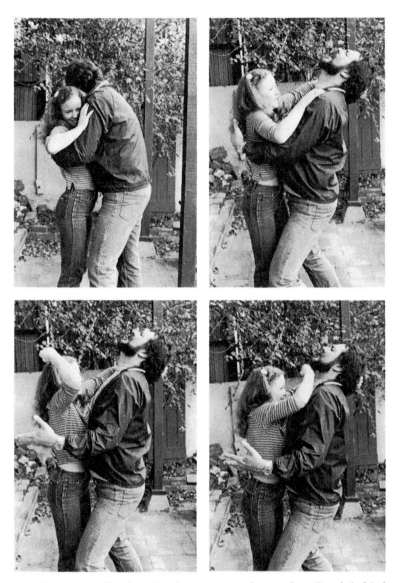

Figure 31: Here's a simple way to mash a masher. Reach behind his head and yank his hair straight down. Then, if you really want to hurt him, use your other hand to hammer on his windpipe.

6. ESCAPES FROM AN UNFRIENDLY EMBRACE

The techniques in this section are especially appropriate for women since it is rare that a man falls victim to a masher or a rapist. Male self-defense students study these techniques so that they can teach them to their female friends, and also in case of a confrontation with a bear-hugging lumberjack who likes to hear vertebrae popping.

I am using the term *embrace* to indicate a far-from-tender encircling of your body by the opponent's arms, in this case exclusively from the front. (Rear embraces are handled differently in a later section.) The nature of this situation dictates that the attacker will grab you in one of two ways. He'll either reach over your arms and pin them to your sides, or he'll grab you around the waist and leave your arms free. In the odd case where only one arm is pinned suitable variations of "arms free" techniques will prove effective.

ATTACK #19

The attacker embraces you from in front (belly to belly), leaving your arms free. This position could represent anything from a drunk trying to steal a kiss from a winsome lass to a carnival weightlifter trying to see how many of your ribs he can snap (because you tried to steal a kiss from his winsome lass . . .).

BASIC DEFENSE #19

This may not seem like much of a basic defense, but the essential key in this situation is simply to keep your wits together. Consider—the idiot left your hands free. There's his head not more than a foot away and you have two free hands. The basic defense is *to remember to use them.*

COUNTERATTACKS FOR SITUATION #19

19-1: This is the point in my class where I like to under-line the differences among karate, judo, and self-defense. Here you are locked in an unwelcome embrace. To escape, a karate student would break the attacker's pelvis with his knee and crack the man's skull with the edge of his hand. A judo student would twist to the side and throw the attacker on the floor, possibly dislocating the man's shoulder or elbow for good measure. But what would a self-defense student do to get loose? What kind of devastatingly effective technique can a poorly trained, out-of-shape self-defense student use to break free from this hold?

Simple. Take your index finger and ram it up his nose. If he doesn't let you go, curl your finger into a hook and yank it out again. He'll let go, all right.

19-2: An option which is far more destructive is to clap your palms smartly over his ears, breaking his eardrums. This must be a very sudden, very forceful double blow which cups the palms directly over the openings of the ear canals. The pain inflicted is so severe that the attacker may actually pass out right before your very eyes. Be aware that you are doing irreparable damage to his ears, so it wouldn't be a tactic to use in fun. Also, it is possible to cause a concussion if your hands meet his head with sufficient force. It isn't much more than a hearty slap, but hitting both sides of the brain case at the same instant puts the blows in opposition to one another and magnifies the effective impact.

19-3: Attack the opponent's eyes. Stick your thumbs in them. Claw at them with your fingernails. Spit in his eyes. Slap your open palms hard over his eyes. Pound on them with your fists. Just remember, it will be sufficient to force him to release his grip in order to protect his eyes. Blinding a man by popping his eyeball with your thumb is an act re-served for times of the greatest desperation.

19-4: If you would like to assault his face with a few

really powerful, clublike blows bring your elbows into play. Snap the front of your bony right elbow across his face (from your right to left), and then smack him with the back of the same elbow on the return trip. Alternate with the left elbow. The odds are that he'll drop you after the first blow when he finds his teeth rattling around inside his mouth like dice in a cup.

19-5: The following technique comes in two flavors, hard and soft. Reach around behind the opponent's head and grasp the hair at the back of his head with your left hand. Yank his hair straight down. This will rock his face back and put his chin in a vulnerable protruding position.

For the soft version, place your right palm under his chin and start to push his head backwards. You will find that your finger tips just about reach his eyes when the heel of your palm is braced under his chin, so why not poke around a little and give him something more to think about? He'll find it a painful and embarrassing position to maintain, and will release you fairly quickly. If he doesn't, use your knee.

The hard version of the technique is to use a powerful palm-heel strike up under his chin, knocking him out and possibly breaking his neck. If you need to kill him (some of my readers are military men) you can just use a right hammer-fist blow to the Adam's apple. It is splendidly exposed when the opponent's head is rotated back like this. (See Figure 31.)

19-6: This one really only works for women. The more macho among us won't even try it.

Throw your arms around the attacker's neck and hug him, pulling yourself up into a cheek-to-cheek position as if in a passionate embrace. (No amorous drunk will suspect that anything is wrong, and the tactic might even lull a would-be rapist momentarily.)

Then suddenly lock your teeth into his ear, lift your feet off the ground, and let go with your arms. You'll drop about two feet and land on your knees, but in the meantime your entire weight will be suspended from the big fellow's dainty little ear. Be ready to block his fists when he lets go of you. He's going to be pretty mad.

87

You can see why male students are reluctant to try this technique. A man just feels inhibited about giving a passionate embrace and ear nibble to some 260-pound lumberjack who is squeezing the life out of him. But look at it this way, gentlemen. What would happen if you were to give that hulking lumberjack a big wet kiss? Would he release you? You bet he would!

ATTACK #20

In situation #19 the key to a successful defense was to remember that your hands were free. In this case *your hands are pinned,* a development which makes most people feel perfectly helpless. You must fight that helpless feeling by reminding yourself that, hands or no hands, your feet are still free. Your knees are free. Your head itself is available as a weapon. And last but not least, those pinned hands are only inches away from the attacker's groin. Remembering these points will be the difference between success and failure when your arms are pinned to your sides.

COUNTERATTACKS FOR SITUATION #20

20-1: Use your legs to throw your body weight from side to side, working your hips backward slightly with each lurch. Soon you will have opened up a wide enough gap to get your palms braced against his hipbones. Lurch and shove until an eighteen-inch gap develops between your pelvis and his. That's when you suddenly dig in with your fingers and yank his hips toward you into your rising knee. For added power, push outward against his hips sharply and watch for his natural reaction to oppose your thrust. As soon as he pushes his hips forward you yank them in toward your knee. This kind of thing is what people mean by the phrase "using the opponent's strength against him."

20-2: Another alternative is to use your head. Tuck your chin down against your chest and rap his face with the top of your forehead. You won't have to hit him very hard to hurt him. While he is concentrating on avoiding getting hit in the teeth, you can pick up one of your feet and

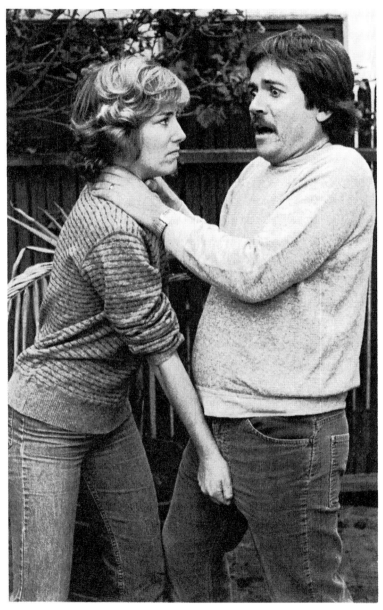

Figure 32: "A bird in the hand . . ."

stomp heavily on his instep, kneecap, or shin.

20-3: There you are, caught in an unfriendly embrace with your hands pinned only inches from his groin. Does that give you any ideas?

One possibility is to make a fist, lock your arm rigidly, bend your knees suddenly, and ram your fist into his groin as your body drops. This groin punch is one of the fastest karate attacks of all due to the extremely short distance your fist has to travel to reach the target. My punch in this situation was once electronically timed at 0.04 second, start to finish. This is five times faster than a normal person can even begin to react.

20-4: Another idea would be to reach in there and grab a fistful of the fellow's most precious possessions. Don't apply any pressure, just get a good snug grip on them. Then look him in the eye and see if he gets the message. He'd have to be pretty stupid not to. (See Figure 32.)

20-5: A variation which works for the ladies is to reach into the fellow's groin and fondle him. (This is a little like putting an alligator to sleep by rubbing his stomach!) He may decide that he's made a lucky catch, until you sort things out, catch a testicle between your thumb and forefinger, and squash it like a ripe grape. Duck and shield your face at the same time. Don't worry about him getting up and running after you. He won't.

7. ATTACKS FROM THE REAR

The coward's standard stock in trade is the surprise attack from behind the victim. Although a blow on the back of the skull gives you little opportunity for retaliation, many muggings begin with a sudden choke, strangle hold, or embrace from the rear instead. If such is the case you can make the mugger wish he had chosen a less hazardous profession.

But the attack from behind is not limited to muggings. Barroom brawls occasionally involve one combatant choking the other from the rear. In the movies, and too often in real life, one thug pins a victim's arms from behind while an accomplice beats him. In all of these situations the ability to speedily dispatch a person who has attacked you from behind could be crucial to your survival.

ATTACK #21

The attacker embraces you from behind, encircling your waist with his arms but leaving your arms free.

BASIC DEFENSE #21

In this position the attacker's arms are fully employed in holding you, and his legs have to be strongly braced to prevent you from pulling him around or overbalancing him. You, on the other hand, have complete freedom of movement with your head, arms, and legs. You can't walk away, it's true, and it is difficult for you to turn around to face your attacker, but otherwise you can do anything. The only portions of the opponent's anatomy that are out of your reach are his back and his groin. His face, hands, legs, and feet are extremely vulnerable.

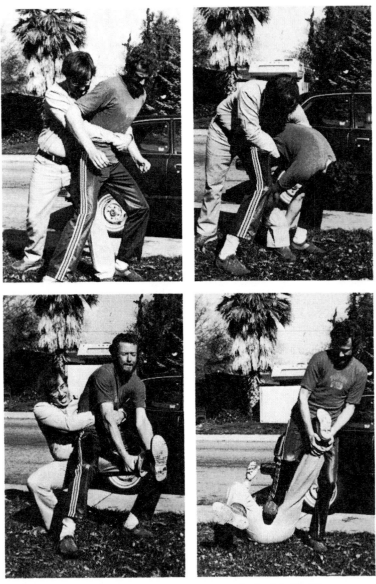

Figure 33: The rear bear hug is easy to deal with. In this sequence the defender performs a basic leg lift on the attacker, and then zeroes in for a crushing stomp to the testicles.

The key defensive principle to remember is that the attacker has immobilized himself by grabbing you this way. There is little that he can do to hurt you without releasing you first. That means you have some time to think before acting. It also means that a second attacker approaching you from the front is by far the more dangerous of the two. Deal with him first.

COUNTERATTACKS FOR SITUATION #21

21-1: The classic trick to pull on someone who is holding you around the waist from behind is to step back and bump into the attacker, knocking him slightly off balance, and then bend sharply at the waist to reach back between your legs and grab one of his ankles with both hands. Straighten up using the strength of your back to yank his foot right up to eye level. (You wind up straddling his leg almost as if you were sitting on his thigh.) (See Figure 33.)

A typical attacker will fall flat on his back as his foot rises above waist level. If you happen to get a limber one, just pick up your feet and let him try to balance both your weight and his own on one foot. (If he can do it, give up!)

Usually the attacker will let go of your waist as he starts to fall, leaving you standing there holding his foot. The fellow's hips land on the ground just behind your feet. For that little something extra, use your heel to stomp backwards into the opponent's groin.

21-2: If you attempt the preceding technique but the attacker does not let go of you as he starts to fall, throw yourself back on top of him so that you land (sit) heavily on his chest or abdomen. He'll wind up with ruptured internal organs or a crushed chest, so don't do this for fun.

If you happen to miss him with your butt (as happens occasionally) immediately shift to a flurry of blows using your elbows, heels, and anything else that becomes available. He'll have to release you to protect himself.

Notice that even in the case of fighting two attackers this technique is still valuable. By throwing yourself backwards to squash the rear assailant you simultaneously drop out of reach of the attacker in front of you. At that point it is best to shift to the techniques described previously for fighting from the ground. Just be sure that you don't bend over to grab one attacker's ankle while the second attacker is within kicking range of your face.

21-3: This technique is similar to 14-2. Take a forceful sudden step out to the right and in the same motion step around behind the attacker with your left foot. Properly executed this move will leave you standing to the right rear of the opponent, with the front of your left hip against his buttocks. Bend forward from the waist and scoop up his knees with your hands.

Straighten your back, lifting his knees straight up. His body will rock back over your left hip and balance there like a teeter-totter. You will find that you can turn him completely upside-down and hold him that way with very little strength or effort. Needless to say, even if you stop here you will have gravely discomfited your opponent.

If embarrassing the opponent is not sufficient to meet the demands of the situation (there might be another attacker to deal with) just bend your knees and fall back as you yank his knees upward. You'll whiplash the back of his skull into the pavement.

21-4: This one is a short, sharp technique for people who don't like the idea of falling on the ground. Look down at your waist where the attacker's hands meet. Grasp his right wrist with your right hand. Using the heel of your left palm, force one of his right finger tips away from you, opposite to its natural direction of bending. You can make this a slow bend, giving him time to let go of you and save his finger, or you can just snap the finger back and break it like a green bean. Either way it will break his hold on your waist.

An appropriate optional finish would be to turn slightly to one side and stomp the sole of your foot back against his knee.

21-5: This is one of the simplest and most effective self-defense techniques, but surprisingly few students discover it spontaneously.

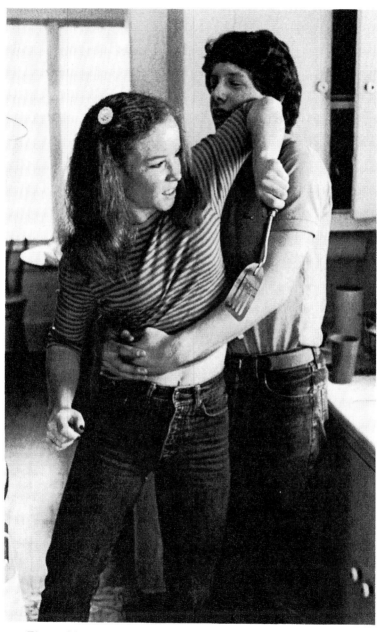

Figure 34: An even simpler solution to the rear bear hug is the classic elbow blow to the jaw. This technique is very simple, very powerful and very effective.

When someone grabs you around the waist from behind (leaving your arms free) all you have to do is twist your body about 90 degrees and smack him in the face with the back of your elbow. If the attacker is too tall to reach with your elbow, use a hammer-fist blow instead. He won't be able to stand up to your blows for long, but in order to escape or retaliate he first must release you, and that was the basic idea anyway. (See Figure 34.)

ATTACK #22

The attacker embraces you from behind, pinning your arms to your sides. This situation is fundamentally similar to attack #21 but your freedom of movement with your hands is greatly diminished.

BASIC DEFENSE #22

This time the attacker has again immobilized himself by using both arms to hold you while bracing for a struggle with both legs. Your legs are still free, but your hands are trapped at your sides.

What can you do in this position?

The key thing to remember is that you are not helpless. For one thing, there are your hands only inches from his groin. The fact that you can also attack his face, legs, and feet seems almost superfluous in comparison. If the idiot wants to pin your hands between his legs, you might as well go ahead and give him what he deserves.

The basic defense in this case is to shift your hips rapidly from side to side, striving to work your hands back behind you into striking position. From this position there are several devastating options.

COUNTERATTACKS FOR SITUATION #22

22-1: Shift your hips to one side, then strike straight back into his groin with a hammer-fist blow. If he blocks the attack by turning his hip in to catch your fist, just shift to the other side. His retreat from your right fist will set him up perfectly for an attack by your left fist.

22-2: Shift your hips to the side. Reach back with one hand and grasp his genitals in your fist. He will probably let go instantly. If not, lock your arm as straight as a ramrod and throw your feet out from under you. Let your weight rip his private parts down to his ankles. (See Figure 35.)

In actual practice it is impossible to maintain a grip tight enough to tear the opponent asunder, but there is a striking "window shade" effect which is sure to get his attention. His genitals stretch down as far as they will go and then pull free of your grip—to snap back into place like a windowshade rolling up. It feels just as sickening as it sounds.

22-3: Here's a variation for those of you who just couldn't bring themselves to perform the previous two techniques. (Teen-age girls sometimes refuse to even pretend to perform the windowshade trick.) Snap your head backward, striking him in the face (nose, lips, and teeth) with the back of your skull. Stomp on his feet and kick back into his knees and shins to distract him with pain. Shift your hips to the side, then drive your elbow straight back into his solar plexus. Mix and match these attacks repetitively until the attacker's grip on you loosens.

As a parting gesture turn around to face him, grab him by the hips and knee him convincingly in the groin.

ATTACK #23

The attacker chokes you with his hands from the rear. Note that this choke is performed with the fingers only, since the attacker's palms and thumbs are appressed to the sides and back of your neck.

DEFENSE AND COUNTERATTACKS
FOR SITUATION #23

23-1: Most self-defense teachers do not cover this attack at all. The few who do tend to rely on the following classic technique. Their confidence is well justified, since there are few other alternatives which a typical self-defense student can work as well.

Reach up to your throat and find the attacker's fingers.

97

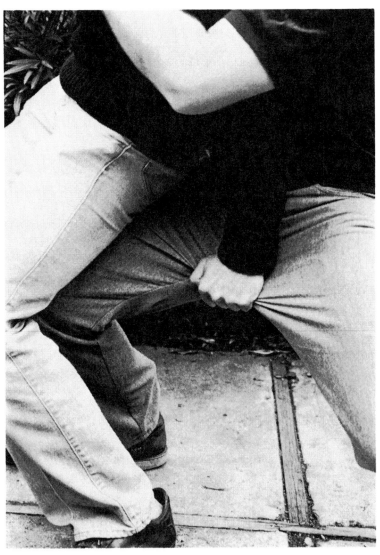

Figure 35: When your arms have been pinned from the rear there are still a few things you can do to ruin the attacker's day. This, the "window shade trick," is one of the best.

Pry and gouge at them until you can get a good grip on one (and only one) finger. The little finger or ring finger is usually the best choice, but take what you can get. (Don't use his thumb.) Snap the finger sideways to break the hold (and the finger).

Do not release his finger. Your firm grip on that dislocated finger will do more to control your assailant than a whole squad of police could do. If you like, you can finish with a kick to the knee or groin before releasing him.

23-2: Another way to break this hold is to bend sharply forward at the waist and turn around to face the attacker, ducking your head under his arm as you turn. Straighten up and finish with a palm-heel strike to the chin, or you can stand up with a forearm wedge technique and counterattack (see basic defense #10).

23-3: Probably the simplest release from this situation, if you are up to it, is to bend forward from the waist and launch a back-kick into the attacker's groin, abdomen or chest. The back-kick might be best described to a layman as a "donkey-kick," in which you lift your knee up to your chest, bend forward, and stomp straight back (horizontally) against the opponent's body. Most men will let go of your neck instantly to avoid a repetition.

23-4: There is another response to this attack which I suggest only to more advanced students, and especially to karate-trained individuals.

Sit down suddenly just behind your heels and roll backward on to your back. As you go down reach up and grasp the attacker's wrists as they twist free from your neck.

He will bend forward in an automatic attempt to follow you down. This leaves you on your back with your head roughly between the attacker's feet. To effect the counterattack, pull down on the attacker's arms while driving the soles of both your feet smartly up under his chin. Properly executed this blow is extremely vicious, and can easily break his neck.

I recommend this technique only to more advanced self-defense students because the roll back and kick must be performed very quickly, with no false moves or wasted motion. Otherwise the frustrated opponent will surely realize that he can stomp on your face, and he will do so. Your defense against this is speed, a commodity which beginners tend to lack.

23-5: Here's an especially effective technique which many people adopt as a favorite. The opponent has grasped your neck from behind as before. Lift your left arm up high as you forcefully turn to your left to face the attacker. Your arm will sweep across over his arms, tearing his hands from your neck. Drop your arm down tightly against your left side to trap his wrists under your armpit. This leaves you with one fist free while he has both wrists trapped. It will take him a moment to get his wits together, so use that right hammer fist quickly in a strike to the temple, side of the neck, or collarbone. (See Figure 36.)

ATTACK #24

The attacker encircles your throat with his right arm, strangling you from behind. This attack is similar to the two chokes described in sections 8-2 and 8-3.

BASIC DEFENSE #24

When you feel someone's arm snaking around your neck from behind, your basic defense is to hunch your shoulders and tuck in your chin. Try to turn your chin into the fold of the opponent's elbow and burrow it in deep. In this way you can keep some of the pressure off your throat. This gives you a little time to think as well as a minor degree of relief from the pain of the attack.

COUNTERATTACKS FOR SITUATION #24

24-1: Grasp his forearm near the elbow with your left hand, and grasp his upper arm near the shoulder with your right hand. Bend sharply at the waist as if to touch your head to your knees, and your opponent will sail right over your head and land on his back. Nine times out of ten he'll release your neck and use his hands to try to break his fall. The

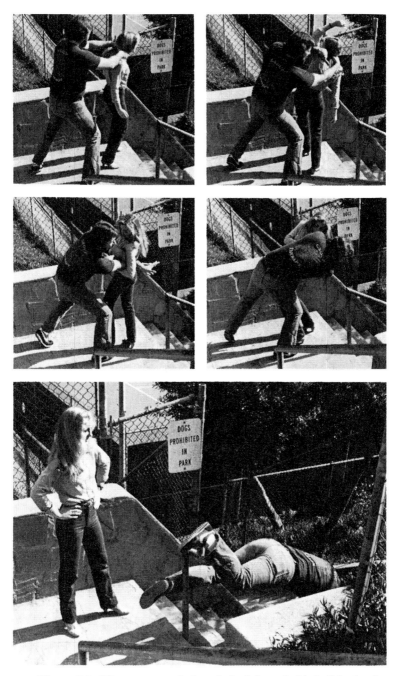

Figure 36: When you are being choked from behind, this simple windmilling spin effectively and reliably turns the tables on the attacker. Of course, a handy stairwell helps.

101

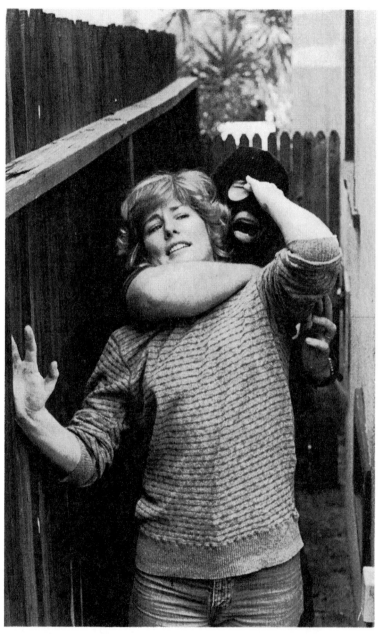

Figure 37: The simplest solution to the strangle hold is a five-fingered stab at the eyes ... which are usually within easy reach.

tenth guy will give your neck a pretty severe twist as he goes over.

A word of caution. Most practice partners you may encounter will gracefully perform a somersault when you use this throw on them, but a few awkward people will just dive straight into the ground headfirst. I nearly killed a student this way one time and the experience has made me very cautious. Usually I refrain from teaching this trick except in the case of the occasional student who is athletically inclined.

24-2: If his body is held straight and stiff so you can't throw him, use a hammer-fist blow to the groin, an elbow into the ribs, and/or a stomp on the foot to loosen him up a little. As soon as he is hurt or distracted, try the throw again.

24-3: Spread and stiffen the fingers of both hands and suddenly stab backwards over both shoulders in search of an unsuspecting eye. In practice just reach back gently and feel for your partner's face. Get used to the idea that you *can* reach his eyes with your fingers from this position. (See Figure 37.)

ATTACK #25

One of the most familiar attacks from the rear is the hammer lock. In this classic attack *the opponent bends your right arm up behind your back* until you writhe in pain. Usually he will grip your arm at the wrist with his right hand. His left hand will either grip your arm, your shoulder or possibly your neck.

BASIC DEFENSE #25

When your right arm is in a hammer lock the basic defense is to bend forward at the waist and twist to your left in an attempt to straighten out your captured arm. By bowing and twisting in this manner you relieve most of the pain. Then you can decide what to do next.

COUNTERATTACKS FOR SITUATION #25

25-1: Use the basic defense to relieve pressure on your arm. After bending forward and twisting to the left, look back at your opponent and use your left leg to stomp at his knee, groin, or abdomen. To magnify the effect, use your captured right hand to grab the opponent's arm as you lean forward. This way you can actually pull him into the kick, and keep him from escaping while you wind up for another kick . . . and another . . . and another . . . .

25-2: Twist sharply to your left until your left shoulder is toward the opponent. As a part of the same motion, use your left hand to deliver a hammer-fist or knife-hand attack to the enemy's temple or neck. Let your arm trail behind your swinging shoulder like a ball on a chain for added power. (See Figure 38.)

25-3: If the attacker uses his left hand to hold your collar or hair so that you cannot bend forward away from him, try twisting to the left and striking the back of his left elbow with the thumb side of your left fist (a ridgehand attack). Another possibility would be to use a hammer-fist or knife-hand attack against his left ribs. The principle is much the same.

25-4: One of the worst possibilities is that the attacker may encircle your neck with his left arm while pressing the hammer lock with his right hand. In this case you will not be able to bow or twist at all. Your only option is to use your feet and your free arm creatively to force him to let you go.

This will be a battle of endurance, since the pressure on your right arm will immediately increase as soon as you try to resist. You must succeed instantly in injuring and distracting him or you will sincerely regret the attempt.

My suggestion is to start with a left hammer fist back into the opponent's groin, followed immediately by a couple of bone-shattering stamps to the instep of the foot. If you are successful he'll release your neck and step back away from you, but he'll probably try to maintain the hammer lock. At that point you should bow, twist and kick as described in technique 24-1.

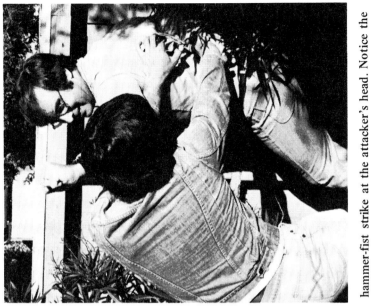

hammer-fist strike at the attacker's head. Notice the subtle touch barely visible in the first photo, where the defender has twisted his hand and trapped the attacker's arm to pull him into the blow.

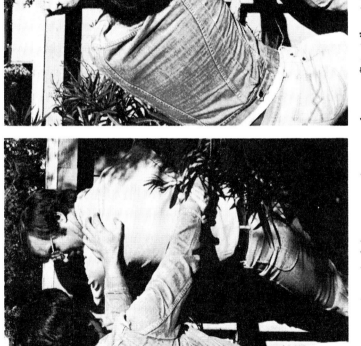

Figure 38: This is the end of the sequence begun in Figure 13. To escape from a hammer lock, twist violently toward your free side and lash out with a

8. DEFENDING AGAINST KNIVES & CLUBS

The subject of weapon defenses is probably the single most controversial topic in the self-defense field. I cringe at some of the published self-defense guides which show how "easy" it is to disarm a knifeman. I can only conclude that the authors just haven't had very much experience sparring with knife duelists. Otherwise they would not be so overconfident on behalf of their readers.

It is essential for a self-defense student to be aware of his own limitations when facing a man who is armed with a knife or club. A stiletto in the hand is easily worth five years of karate training, a fact which scores of karate students have given their lives to prove. I do show my self-defense students how to disarm a knife or club fighter, but I only present these techniques to prove that most people cannot make them work. In my experience a self-defense student has about one chance in twenty of defeating such a person without getting killed in the process. When confronting a weapon the only safe course is to escalate, to produce a more powerful weapon. I prefer a .45 automatic!

There is another dangerous misconception about disarming techniques which is almost never mentioned in self-defense books. This is the fact that military hand-to-hand combat manuals sometimes show techniques which just don't work, apparently in an attempt to raise the morale of boot-camp trainees. This is a psychological effort to convince disarmed soldiers to keep fighting in spite of the odds—an admirable quality in an army but stupid in the street. Don't be taken in. Read those military manuals with more than a little skepticism. You must *never use real weapons in practice!* Use rubber knives and plastic baseball bats—never the real thing. It's far too easy to kill your practice partner otherwise.

ATTACK #26

The attacker holds the knife point down like an icepick with the sharp edge facing inward toward himself. *He then raises the knife over his head and stabs downward toward your chest.* This attack is the classic way in which an ignorant person handles a knife. It usually, but not always, implies that the attacker is naive and may fall for one of the simpler defensive techniques. It may also mean that the attacker is sophisticated and is trying to deceive you. It's a dangerous business.

The following discussion will also apply to situations where the attacker is swinging a short club down at your head. In general the defensive moves are about the same, but there are differences which will be noted where appropriate.

BASIC DEFENSE #26

Starting with either foot, and making the first step in any appropriate direction, run for your life! Unless there is some vital circumstance which prevents flight the best defensive tactic is to run away. Knives and clubs are terrible weapons which most people do not respect sufficiently. A knifeman can kill you every bit as dead as a gunman and almost as quickly. Don't be a fool. Live to fight another day.

Now that the sensible advice is out of the way we'll get down to the terrifying possibility that you cannot flee. Your pregnant wife is with you. She's holding your two-year-old daughter in her arms. Your aged mother is cowering behind you. Flight is out of the question. You must stand your ground and protect them. Now what do you do?

First you utter a silent prayer that your wife will have the sense to help you and not just stand there shrieking hysterically like they do in the movies. If she just throws a bag of dirty diapers in the attacker's face or starts whipping him over the head with her coat you will have a good chance of coming out of this alive. One outrageous tactic is to throw the baby in the attacker's arms. I know that there isn't a mother in the world who could actually *do* it, but think of the look on the knifer's face!

The basic defense when meeting this attack is to step backward and to your left with your right foot in an attempt to pivot your body out of the path of the descending blade. That way you may survive even if you fail to block or parry the weapon. We'll examine three counterattacks from this posture.

COUNTERATTACKS FOR SITUATION #26

26-1: First I want to describe the classic response to this attack as taught in many military manuals. As the attacker steps in to stab, perform the basic defense by taking a long step back and to the left with your right foot. Use an "X" up-block to catch his forearm and block the attack. An "X" block consists of crossing your right wrist over your left wrist, palms down, and raising your arms over your head to meet the attacker's descending forearm *(not the knife!)*. If all goes well you will trap the attacker's wrist in the top of the "X" between your wrists. (If all does *not* go well you get the point of the knife stuck in the top of your skull.)

Assuming that you have been successful with the block— not a small assumption—the next step is to grasp his forearm with your right hand and pull it down past your hip, twisting his arm to bring the back of the elbow up as you do so. With a little experimentation you will find that this is a simple, natural, and powerful motion. Finish by using a left hammer-fist attack to the back of his elbow to dislocate the joint and force him to drop the knife.

I have a couple of comments about this technique. The first is that you should only attempt it against a total fool who happens to be both drunk and blind. Most self-defense students can't make a strong enough "X" block to stop the downward plunge of the knife anyway, and even if they could the block leaves them wide open for a disembowling

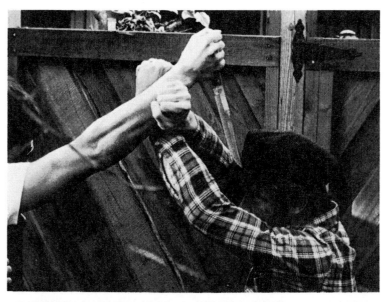

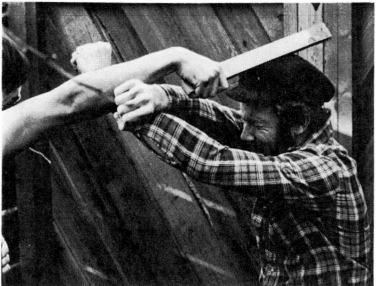

Figure 39: Here are two examples of how not to use the "X" up-block. No matter what the military manuals say, knives and clubs come right through it!

stroke if the first attack was a fake.

On the other hand when the "X" block is properly executed it is extremely effective. I can speak from bitter experience. One time I was playing the part of the attacker when a very serious student really let me have it with an "X" block. There was a loud snap, the knife dropped to the floor, and we all looked with amazement at the new bend that had appeared in my arm. Incidentally, we were both wearing protective padding on our arms at the time, the kind some people now use for full contact karate practice. The only effect of the padding was to lead us into using dangerous amounts of force during practice.

If you try this technique against a club you'll discover a very disconcerting fact. When you use the "X" block to stop the attackers downward swing, his forearm stops but his wrist just bends and the club comes right on down to rap you on the head. This effect is almost guaranteed to occur whether the attacker intends to do it or not. I know this from repeated experiences with practice partners who didn't really intend to hit me, but did. Don't be taken in by self-defense books which confidently suggest using the "X" block against a club. (See Figure 39.)

26-2: For those of you who like flashy knife defenses that don't necessarily work, there is a variation on technique 26-1 which will amuse you. Perform the basic defense, block, grab and pull as described above. Then, instead of using the hammer-fist attack on his elbow, turn to your right and pass your left arm over his upper arm. Grasp his wrist with both hands as you trap his upper arm under your armpit (effecting a straight arm lock). In this position you can put pressure on his shoulder and elbow by levering his wrist upward. Hold his wrist up high, throw your feet out from under you, and hang your whole weight on his shoulder to smack his head into the pavement. (Notice the similarity to technique 11-3.)

This is a very dramatic finish which seems "to serve him right," but don't get too attached to it. Remember that in order to get this far you first have to work the minor miracle of catching his arm during the initial attack. Otherwise it will be you on the pavement. Good luck.

26-3: The response I favor in this situation isn't very dramatic but it has the virtue of working pretty well. As the attacker steps in with knife upraised, perform the basic defense to get your body out of the path of the blade. Use your left hand to slap-block the attacker's arm (not the knife) to your right, which simply knocks the knife (or club) a little farther away as it passes.

In the split second before he can recover his wits and launch a second attack he will be vulnerable. Be alive to any chance to stomp on the attacker's right knee with your left foot at this time. Your relative positions won't always work out correctly for this kick, but if circumstances permit all you have to do is rock back on your right foot, lift your left leg, and stomp down to rip apart the ligaments that hold his knee joint together. Then you can walk away as slowly as you like.

If this approach doesn't seem to fit the situation shift into the general defense advocated later in this chapter.

26-4: There is a fun variation of the previous technique with which more advanced students like to experiment. As the knife or club attack comes in toward your upper body, sidestep and slap the attacker's wrist to the right as before. This time, however, use your hand to grab his wrist and ride it down. By adding your downward force to his own, you can encourage the attacker to stab himself in the groin or thigh. If he is using a club he winds up whacking his knee. Either way he deserves it. This trick requires timing and confidence on the part of the defender, but beyond that it is not especially difficult to perform. (See Figure 40.)

ATTACK #27

During a knife holdup, *the attacker holds the knife in his right hand with the point at your throat.* He grips the knife like a fencing foil, and seems to delight in shoving it in your face to see you flinch. This kind of behavior is fairly common among teen-aged terrors whose confidence in their

112

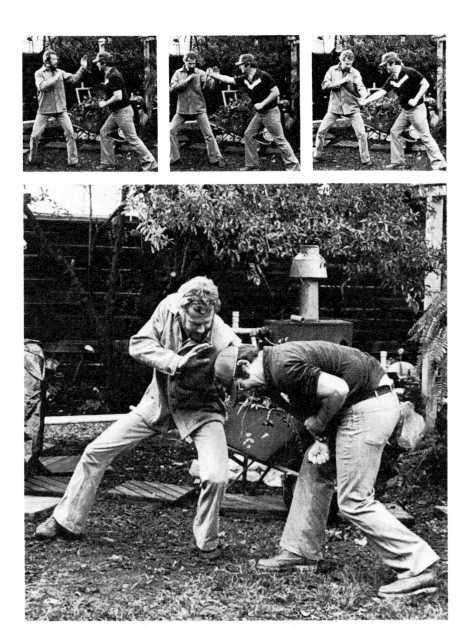

Figure 40: If you have good timing and a lot of nerve you can convert an overhand knife attack into a devastating surprise for the attacker. This is one of the techniques which works better in real life than in practice because of the power which a real assailant puts into the attack.

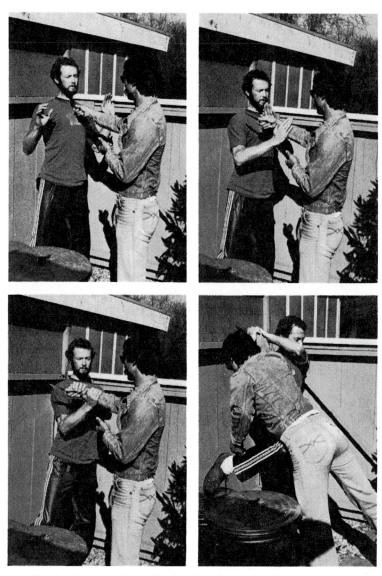

Figure 41: One of the few knife defenses which really work is this response to a hold up. The slapping motion shown in the second photo usually breaks the attacker's grip and sends the knife spinning to the ground, but if not there is always the knee.

own manhood is not very great. Alternately, you can sometimes provoke a more cautious robber into this kind of behavior by judicious insults. Of course, that can also get you killed.

BASIC DEFENSE #27

The basic defense in this situation is to raise your hands in the classic "hands up" posture, but hold them no higher than your head. Now take a look at the attacker's hand. If he is holding the knife so that the point almost touches your throat or face you have a respectable chance of disarming him without getting hurt. If he's holding the knife farther away the odds are against you.

The following technique is best applied when the attacker's attention has been distracted a little, but in many cases even average students can perform the trick faster than the opponent can react, distraction or not. Bring your hands together hard in a clapping motion, catching the back of his fist with the palm of your left hand and striking the inside of his wrist with the palm of your right hand. If you succeed in bending his wrist in toward the inside of his forearm it will involuntarily open and release the knife.

This is one of the few knife disarming techniques which actually seems to work well enough for me to recommend it without conscience pangs. If you can just tease the robber into raising the blade to your face you can clap your hands on his fist and disarm him faster than he can react. Unfortunately, not all knife-bearing attackers are content to threaten before attacking, nor are they stupid enough to hand the weapon to you on a silver platter like this. But just in case you get lucky, this one seems to work now and then.

COUNTERATTACKS FOR SITUATION #27

27-1: Use either your left or right hand to deliver a knife-hand chop to the attacker's throat, or a hammer-fist attack to his temple. Executed with enough force these attacks can be lethal. You don't mess around with a guy who is threatening your life.

27-2: Here's a risky back-up technique in case your initial clap doesn't knock the knife out of his hand. If you fail to bend his wrist far enough to make his hand open up you'll probably wind up holding his fist in your hands. Quickly shift your grip so that both of your thumbs are on the back of his fist and your fingers curl around either side toward his palm. This is similar to technique 11-2. Now pull his hand toward you with your fingers, press it away from you with your thumbs (putting painful pressure on the wrist joint), and twist his hand violently to your left. If everything works he'll drop the knife and fall on his right shoulder.

This technique is fun to practice but heaven help you if you ever really need it. I just can't see that mythical attacker standing still and allowing you to play with his fist like that. All he has to do is rip his arm back out of your grip before you get the hold applied and he'll be free—and you'll lose a couple of fingers in the process. Not a good situation.

27-3: As an alternative to 27-2 I suggest the following counterattack. If you didn't succeed in disarming him with the clap just let your hands get a good tight grip on his arm instead. Your right hand in particular can get a powerful grip on his wrist, and your left hand can obtain a less effective grip on the back of his fist. Note that this does not involve fumbling around for new holds after the clap. Your hands just grab whatever they catch.

With this two-handed grip established the attacker will have a much harder time yanking his hand out of your control. Be assured that he will try, however, and that his whole attention will momentarily reside on getting his knife hand free. This is your opportunity.

Yank his hand to the side over your right shoulder as you step in slightly to the left of him with your left foot. He'll never see your right knee coming up. (He'll feel it, though.) (See Figure 41.)

ATTACK #28

The following techniques are for any time *someone threatens you with a knife or club* in any way, but particu-

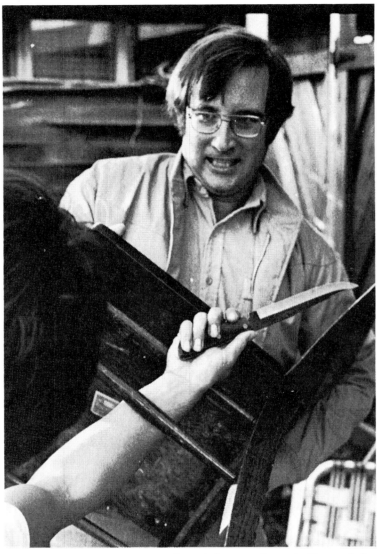

Figure 42: The best expedient defense against a knife attack is a straight-backed wooden chair. It is every bit as effective as it looks.

larly for those times when the attacker really seems to know what he is doing. This section contains a miscellaneous collection of techniques which have seemed more effective than most. One of them might save your life.

BASIC DEFENSES #28

28-1: Don't wait for him to attack! Sling things at his legs—lamps, stools, garbage can lids, fire irons, chairs, golf clubs—anything in reach that can hurt his legs and slow him down. If you can reduce his mobility enough, you may be able to walk away in safety.

28-2: Don't wait for him to attack! Pick up a light chair and rush him with it, lion-tamer fashion. Aim one foot of the chair at his throat and the opposite foot at his groin. The seat of the chair serves as a very reliable shield to protect you from the knife. Remember to thrust or charge with the legs of the chair. Don't make the TV mistake of swinging the chair like an axe or club. (See Figure 42.)

This technique is remarkably effective against a knife, partly because the chair serves as both an offensive and defensive weapon and partly because very few knifemen have ever confronted an opponent with a chair. It disconcerts them, to say the least. Against a club it's better to use the chair primarily as a shield and kick under it at his legs and groin. This defense is highly recommended.

28-3: Use a book, purse, pillow, or coat as a shield by holding it stretched tightly between your hands with your arms fully extended in front of you. After a little practice you will find that it is remarkably easy to block all kinds of attacks using such a simple shield. Incidentally, the block does not have to intercept the knife. Blocking his wrist or forearm is easier and is just as effective. (For the club it's better to block the hand and base of the club rather than the forearm, and best to catch it right at the beginning of the swing.) Be alert to any opportunity to deliver an incapacitating kick to his knee or groin.

This technique of blocking a knife or club attack works best during the first few lunges, but after that an opponent will back off a little and try to get clever. You'll see the difference. Once he gets his wits together he'll feint with a false attack to draw your block, then he'll shift suddenly to another attack. If you're quick you'll be able to frustrate even this approach, but sooner or later the attacker will realize that he can grab your shield with his free hand. If he succeeds you must instantly—*instantly*—release the shield. If you follow your instincts and try to pull back on the shield he'll kill you for sure.

This is a very effective defense and is highly recommended.

28-4: Possibly the best way to meet a weapon attack is to fall flat on your back and use your feet to fight off the attacker. This puts your most vulnerable vital areas out of reach of the opponent's weapon hand, and puts your best-protected area (your feet inside your shoes) between you and the weapon.

Fight the standing opponent from the ground as described earlier in the book but be very aggressive, scuttling in at him and kicking viciously at his knees and shins. Yell loudly and fiercely to distress the attacker and to summon aid. Don't be afraid to take a few shallow cuts across the bony part of the shin if necessary in order to get within striking distance of his knees. Club blows across the shins are to be avoided, however! When he swings at your legs counter by kicking directly at the inside of his wrist. You won't get more than one good chance to break his arm this way so make it a good one.

This tactic is so unusual that even very experienced attackers are likely to be taken aback by it. (In fact, they may collapse in laughter.) Try it out with your practice partner. You'll be amazed at how well the tactic works.